The Complete Home Encyclopedia of
FOOD MIRACLES

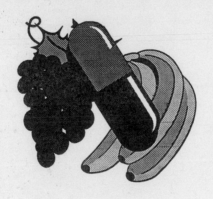

The Complete Home Encyclopedia of
FOOD MIRACLES

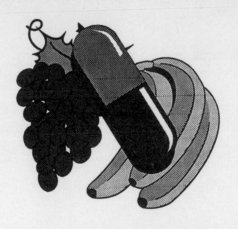

William H. Lee, PhD
Stephen Langer, MD and James F. Scheer
David A. Keiper

Instant Improvement, Inc.

Instant Improvement, Inc.
210 East 86th Street
New York, New York 10028

Manufactured in the United States of America

The Complete Home Encyclopedia of Food Miracles
ISBN 0-941683-05-2

ABOUT THE AUTHORS

Doctor William H. Lee, R.Ph., Ph.D., is a master herbalist, a registered pharmacist, and has his doctorate in nutrition. He has written numerous books and articles for the professional health field, as well as for the general public. He is the author of *The Question and Answer Book of Vitamins*, *Herbs and Herbal Medicine*, *The Medical Benefits of Mushrooms*, *Pre-Menstrual Syndrome*, *The Vitamin Robbers*, and many more. His monthly column, *On Nutrition*, appears in American Druggist Magazine.

* * * * *

Stephen Langer, M.D., is President of *The American Nutritional Medical Association*. He practices Preventive Medicine and Clinical Nutrition in Berkeley, California. He is Consulting Editor of the *National Examiner*, and the author, with James F. Scheer, of *Solved: The Riddle of Illness*.

James F. Scheer has authored or co-authored fourteen books, most of them in the fields of health and nutrition. He has edited two health publications: *Let's Live* and *Food-Wise*, and some twelve hundred of his articles have been published by various magazines.

* * * * *

David A. Keiper graduated from Cornell University in 1953 with a degree in Engineering Physics, with emphasis on mathematics, physics, and engineering. He later had four years of graduate studies at the University of Pennsylvania, in zoology, physiology, molecular biology, biophysics, and biochemistry. His career as a research scientist has been divided between applied physics and medical biophysics.

IMPORTANT NOTICE

This book contains material for informational and educational purposes only. It seeks to make people aware of their health needs.

If any person makes a decision to use any data found in this book, the decision rests completely with that person and his or her own doctor.

This book is not a substitute for personal medical supervision by a qualified health professional. People with health problems should consult with their physician.

Any action taken by the reader concerning therapies or individual substances rests solely with the reader and his or her doctor.

TABLE OF CONTENTS

HOW TO DEVELOP A SKY HIGH I.Q.

by Stephen Langer, M.D. and James F. Scheer

HOW TO DEVELOP A SKY HIGH I.Q.

You can become a genius by the time you finish reading this chapter and applying its simple information.

An extravagant promise?

See for yourself as the lines on these pages march before your eyes.

Consider the work of Professor Robert Rivera, who regularly lofts Intelligence Quotients (I.Q.s) of students from the average level — 110 to 120 — by as much as thirty points, into the genius class.

Rivera doesn't do it with magic or mirrors, just with uncommonly uncommon common sense. A memory expert and speech teacher at Valley College in Van Nuys, California, Rivera knows well a basic fact of life and physiology.

More efficient blood flow and oxygen circulation to the brain are the major rocket boosters for the I.Q. Just about any aerobic exercise done for fifteen or twenty minutes will rev up the ability to think and remember more efficiently, but Professor Rivera does it the easy way — with two simple exercises which bring phenomenal results within minutes!

Rich Returns With Rivera Routines

His students like to use them regularly before quizzes and final exams, because they bring a major I.Q. takeoff. Businessmen and women, too, use them before critical meetings or writing difficult reports or proposals.

Here's how they're done.

Inhale for eight counts. Hold your breath for twelve counts, then slowly exhale for ten counts. Rivera advises repeating this exercise ten times. He warns that if you begin to feel dizzy, stop right away.

For the second exercise, stand and flatten yourself against a wall, then stretch upward. Do this ten times. Some people practice both routines and experience a major I.Q. takeoff. Rivera also advises sitting up straight at the desk for maximum brain efficiency. A bowed back and round shoulders reduce blood circulation to the brain.

Do the Rivera routines several times daily, and you'll always be at the Mount Everest peak of your ability to think.

"Geniuses have better blood flow to the brain," Rivera told the writers.[1]

The Importance of Being Oxygenized

All right, geniuses and geniuses on the way, why is oxygen to the brain so vital? Simple. Like all the rest of us, the brain needs energy to run. That energy comes from a "burning" of glucose, the brain's major fuel. And it can't happen without oxygen, just as your car engine can't fire without oxygen. With limited oxygen, the burning slows down and, along with it, thinking and remembering.

Although your brain weighs in at about two percent of your body weight, it attracts and uses about twenty-five percent of the oxygen you inhale. Each hour your brain uses up about a teaspoonful of glucose.

In his book, *The New Psychiatry*, Nathan Masor, M.D., verifies that the grey matter, where thinking takes place, uses as much as 25 percent of your oxygen intake.[2] Blood in the arteries of your brain must have an oxygen saturation of 90 percent for efficient thinking, he states. If it is just five percent less (85 percent), your ability for fine concentrating and carrying on precise muscle coordination decreases. Cut the oxygen saturation down to 74 percent and you start making faulty judgments and decisions. You become emotionally unstable and your nervous system becomes depressed. Starve yourself of oxygen for four minutes and you may suffer irreversible brain damage.[3]

Why Too Little Oxygen Is Delivered

Other than physical inactivity, the major causes for sluggish and/or impaired blood circulation, with insufficient blood delivered to the brain, are anemia, too low thyroid function, or narrowed arteries.

All anemias — iron-deficiency, pernicious, and megalo-blastic — have something in common: they limit the delivery of the needed amounts of oxygen to your body's trillions of cells, including those of the brain.

Let's get specific about iron-deficiency anemia, because it is by far the most widespread type. Over and above its symptoms of fatigue and exhaustion, typical of all anemias, iron-deficiency anemia brings on low attention span, breathlessness after exertion, brittle nails, headaches, gastrointestinal upset, pale skin, rapid pulse and, sometimes, loss of sexual desire.

This anemia is caused by the body's need for more iron, a deficiency that can result from loss of blood, repeated pregnancies, or the body's inability to absorb enough iron.

Iron intake and absorption are key to correcting this condition because this mineral, along with protein and copper, makes up hemoglobin in red blood cells, those micro freight cars that carry oxygen to the brain and elsewhere.

Groups most likely to be iron-deficient are menstruating women, teenagers, repeatedly pregnant women and older individuals. Numerous studies show that at least 200 to 500 mg of vitamin C daily — you can't get that much from diet alone — help you absorb iron more effectively, no matter what your age.[4]

Low Thyroid, Low Oxygen

Low thyroid function can deprive you of oxygen in a different way than do the various anemias. A featherweight, coral-colored bow-tie of a gland, semi-circling the windpipe under the Adam's apple, the thyroid is small but mighty. Your five quarts of blood circulate through it once an hour, bringing iodide, the substance the thyroid gland needs to make hormones, and picking up the thyroid hormone to drop off at each cell for its use.

Too little thyroid hormone, causing the condition called hypo-thyroidism (low thyroid function), makes the brain and body motors run sluggishly. You can expect only limited service from brain and body if you are hypothyroid. (Later on, we'll show you how you can test yourself to find out.)

The late Louis Berman, M.D., an internationally known endocrinologist, sums up the importance of full thyroid function:

"Without thyroid, there can be no complexity of thought, no learning, no education, no habit formation, no responsive energy for situations, as well as no physical unfolding of faculty function. No reproduction of kind with no sign of adolescence at expected age and no exhibition of sex tendencies thereafter."[5]

What it all adds up to is that with no thyroid gland, we would be vegetables, human rutabagas. All right, but where does too little oxygen delivery come in?

In hypothyroids, heartbeat slows, blood pressure drops, circulation loses its needed vigor (especially noticeable in cold hands and feet and low energy). Thinking is slow and memory is, at best, undependable.

Low thyroid function also shows in lazy blood circulation, causing a too slow delivery of oxygen and glucose to brain and body cells, and a decreasing of the rate at which food is burned in the cells (by limiting the amount of red blood cells that can be made — remember red blood cells carry oxygen), thereby raising blood cholesterol levels and contributing to atherosclerosis (narrowing of arteries), which further cuts down on oxygen and nutrient deliveries.

Nathan Masor states that any narrowing of the key brain arterioles, by even a sixteenth of an inch, can limit the amount of oxygen that gets through, to the point of lowering mental efficiency and bringing on emotional disturbances. (More about this later and how to cope with it naturally.)

Hypothyroidism: How Widespread?

In, *Solved: The Riddle of Illness* (Keats Publishing, Inc.), the authors offered evidence that perhaps 40 percent of the population suffers from undetected hypothyroidism, because this ailment often escapes detection by conventional blood tests (the only ones on which orthodox doctors rely).[6]

These conventional tests may be specific for this ailment, but they are not usually sensitive enough to reveal it, a fact that numerous researchers in recent years have found to be true. For real accuracy, the no-cost, do-it-yourself Barnes Basal Temperature Test, the armpit test, has proved to be a far more reliable indicator of low thyroid function.

At one time it was mentioned in the Journal of the American Medical Association and in the Physicians Desk Reference (the PDR), but now orthodox medicine tries to ignore it, probably because there's no money in it for physicians or labs. Its originator, Broda O. Barnes, M.D., Ph.D, an internationally recognized thyroid gland authority, found a common denominator in hypothyroidism: subnormal temperature.

This is how to use the test, as described in our book, *Solved: The Riddle of Weight Loss*. (Healing Arts, Press, 1989):

"On the night before the test, shake down an oral thermometer and leave it on your bedside table. The very moment you wake up after a good night's sleep — no alcohol the night before, please — stay in bed and place the thermometer firmly in the armpit, leaving it there for ten minutes. (Do not take your temperature by mouth! Although mouth and armpit temperatures are identical under ideal circumstances, sore throats, colds and sinusitis raise oral temperature, making for a false reading.)

"If your reading is lower than 97.8 — normal resting temperature is 97.8 to 98.2 — even if just a fraction below, you are very likely hypothyroid. Repeat the process the next morning. If you are a woman of child-bearing years, perform the test only on the second and third days of menstruation."

Alternative doctors recognize the validity of this test and health food store owners usually know the names of an alternative physician in their area.

First generation hypothyroids can often correct the condition with a daily kelp tablet, which is rich in iodine, the thyroid gland's main nutrient.

Second generation hypothyroids, and beyond, need to have thyroid hormone prescribed. The preference in my practice is Armour, a natural desiccated thyroid, rather than a synthetic.

Too Low Body Temperature
Undermines Thinking

A giant reason for coping successfully with low thyroid function is that hypothyroids have a subnormal temperature which subtly sabotages ability to think.

Psychologist Emanuel Donchin and electrophysicist Noel K. Marshall, of the University of Illinois' Cognitive Psychophysiology Laboratory, made a significant discovery not long ago. Small daily changes in body temperature — one to two degrees under normal — reduced certain types of brain responses in tested human subjects.[7]

Even slightly depressed body temperatures impair our higher thought processes and slow down our movements. Although we may not be aware of it, our brains react more slowly.

In hypothermia (subnormal temperature) measurable brain wave peaks are markedly delayed. However, when temperatures are brought up to normal, brain waves also speed up and normalize.

Brain wave reactions to subnormal body temperature are so similar to those manifested in brain damage that the researchers urge doctors diagnosing similar cases to first rule out low body temperature before concluding that a patient has irreversible brain damage.

Research results of Donchin and Marshall parallel those of G.A. Kerkhof and associates at the University of Leiden in the Netherlands, who found that body temperatures definitely influence the brain in a manner that determines how test subjects rate their performance of sundry tasks.[8]

Another fascinating discovery of the Kerkhof team was that there's good reason why some of us say, "I'm a morning person," or "I'm an evening person". We do our best and most efficient work at one of these times and with good reason: peak performance coincides with normal temperatures, and lesser performance with subnormal temperatures. Ability to concentrate for long, long periods goes right along with normal temperatures.

Individuals with the low temperatures of hypothyroidism, often one to two and a half degrees below normal, suffer a severe handicap, whether on the production line or in the executive suite — symptoms such as slow-motion response, poor coordination and accident-proneness, slower mental processes and impaired memory.

Foods That Skyrocket Your I.Q.

A number of rat studies show that undernourished rats have a tougher time thinking their way through a maze than well-nourished rats.

Various tests have shown that rats need a minimum of 12 1/2 micrograms of vitamin B-1 daily, among other nutrients, to be well nourished. In one experiment, when given only three micrograms of this vitamin daily, they were slow getting through a maze. However, when fed 100 micrograms, they hurried through in record time.[9]

That's great if you're a rat, but how does this relate to us?

About the same, as numerous studies show.

Here's a "for instance".

In one study, intelligence of well-nourished children was compared with that of undernourished children. All efforts were made to match the test subjects, eliminating such factors as difference of parents' intelligence.[10]

Results surprised even the investigators. The well-nourished children scored an amazing 22.6 points higher in I.Q. than the undernourished ones.

A Striking Experiment

One of the most dramatic demonstrations of a vitamin boosting ability to think effectively was the study of Dr. Ruth Flinn Harrell at the Presbyterian Children's Home in Lynchburg, Virginia.[11] The vitamin was B-1 and Dr. Harrell stumbled upon the idea of making the study by a mixture of curiosity and sharp observation.

She had noted a strange and unexpected change in a young man, an accident victim, at Johns Hopkins Hospital. Suffering from an aphasia, the loss of ability to speak or write, the victim was going through a long and tedious process of reeducation. Then, suddenly, he began learning so rapidly that he was cured and returned to his old job.

Dr. Harrell examined and analyzed the case records to find out why the unexpected spurt in ability to learn and the only reason she could discover was this: for half a dozen days before the dramatic recovery, the patient had been given a low potency vitamin B-1 pill with a meal.

Rats and People Respond

Dr. Harrell compared white rat's ability to solve difficult mazes, first with vitamin B-1 added to their diets, then with none, and she found that the B-1 boosts got the rats through the mazes much more rapidly.

Results encouraged Dr. Harrell to try the same vitamin on three children so mentally handicapped that they could not learn to speak. On a daily vitamin B-complex tablet, all three showed a marked ability to learn, and two actually learned to speak and then could live like normal children.

These preliminaries led to the main event. Dr. Harrell next tested to see if a small amount of vitamin B-1 added to the daily diet would influence the ability to learn and enhance various skills. Over a six week period, in a double-blind study of paired children of matched ability — ages 9 to 19 — one group was given two milligrams of vitamin B-1 and the others were given a look-alike placebo. The children who received the vitamin scored from 7 to 87 percent higher in mental ability and physical skills than those who got the placebo, leading Dr. Harrell to conclude that a certain nutritional state of the nervous system has to be reached for effective learning.

And the experiments of two separate researchers reinforced her conclusion. Bruno Minz in the Laboratory of the Sorbonne University in Paris announced in 1938 that a cut nerve leaked a fluid containing vitamin B-1 and, also, that when a nerve was electrically stimulated, it gave off 80 times more vitamin B-1 than a nerve at rest.[12]

A year later, R.R. Williams announced that many of the impulses passing through a nerve fiber change that fiber chemically so it must be constantly supplied with new nutrients through the process of metabolism (fuel burning). And vitamin B-1 seems to be the spark plug that ignites this fuel burning process.[13]

The Vitamin B-1 Brain Crisis

Most Americans are short-changing their minds — bodies, also — and reducing themselves to second-rate thinkers by taking in too little vitamin B-1.

Test yourself to see if you're sabotaging your mind:

1. Do you eat white bread and refined cereals regularly?
2. Do you put sugar on your cereals and eat candy, cookies, donuts or sweet rolls every day?
3. Do you have one or more alcoholic drinks daily without taking a vitamin B supplement, including vitamin B-1?
4. Do you smoke regularly?
5. Do you cook most of your vegetables?
6. Do you eat raw fish frequently?
7. Do you drink two or more cups of coffee daily?
8. Are you on the pill, pregnant or nursing?
9. Do you take antacids after one or more daily meals?
10. Are you stressed on the job, at home, or with a chronic physical ailment, anxiety or depression?
11. Do you take estrogen or sulfa drugs?

If you answered "yes" to three or more of the above, you are probably vitamin B-1 deficient — the more "yesses", the more acute the deficiency.

Food supplements and the foods richest in vitamin B-1, in milligrams for slightly less than four ounces, are:

brewer's yeast, 16	buckwheat and oats, 0.60
torula yeast, 15	hazelnuts, 0.46
sunflower seeds, 2.2	rye, 0.43
wheat germ, 2.0	lentils and corn, 0.37
royal jelly, 1.5	brown rice, 0.34
pine nuts, 1.3	walnuts, 0.33
peanuts, 1.2	egg yolk, 0.32
soybeans, 1.10	chickpeas, 0.31
sesame seeds, 0.98	blackstrap molasses, 0.28

brazil nuts, 0.96   liver, 0.25
bee pollen, 0.93   almonds, 0.25
pecans, 0.86   barley and salmon, 0.21
alfalfa and peas, 0.80   eggs, 0.17
millet, 0.73   lamb and mackerel, 0.15
beans, 0.68

Over and above vitamin B-1 rich foods, some of my patients wish to guarantee themselves maximum brain power by taking a vitamin B-1 supplement. However, I recommend that they take a vitamin B-complex tablet or capsule containing at least 50 milligrams (mg) of the main B fractions daily, because taking individual B vitamins can sometimes cause imbalances.

Of course, the B-complex tablet or capsule works better if you eat mainly whole grain cereals and bread, raw or lightly cooked vegetables, minimize or eliminate coffee, alcohol and smoking, and learn to handle stress before it manhandles you — that is, accepting stressors as challenges with which you can cope, rather than as depressants or frustrations with which you can't cope.

Vitamin C Gets Into The Act

Vitamin C is well-known for promoting healthy gums, teeth, bones and blood vessels, for shortening the duration of colds, for wound-healing, and for strengthening the immune system, but few individuals know it has also been found helpful in boosting the I.Q.

One study revealed that matched students with higher blood serum levels of vitamin C had an almost five point higher I.Q. than those with a lower blood level of this vitamin. This doesn't sound like much of a gain, but the researchers found it statistically significant.[14] Then both groups were given additional vitamin C — a glass of orange juice daily for six months. The group which had shown superior I.Q. level gained only 2/100ths of a point, but the other group gained 3.54 points.

Supplements and foods containing the most vitamin C, in milligrams per units of just under four ounces, are:

rose hips, 3,000
acerola cherries, 1,100
guavas, 240
black currants, 200
parsley, 170
green peppers, 110
watercress, 80
chives, 70
strawberries, 55
persimmons, 52
spinach, 51
oranges, 50
cabbage, 47
squash, 22

grapefruit, 38
papaya, 37
elderberries and kumquats, 36
dandelion greens
  and lemons, 35
cantaloupe, 33
green onions, 32
limes, 31
mangoes, 27
tangerines and tomatoes, 23
romaine lettuce and
  raspberries, 21
loganberries, 24

Glutamic Acid and Grey Matter

On the hunch that glutamic acid, an amino acid derived from whole wheat, soy beans or beet roots, might be one of the few nutrients "burned up" by brain cells and might, therefore, boost brain function, three researchers at the Columbia College of Physicians and Surgeons fed concentrated amounts of it to rats. They found that those rats on the supplement thought their way through a maze twice as fast as those not given the glutamic acid.

Then, Drs. Zimmerman, Burgemeister, and Putnam experimented to see if this nutrient would rev up the I.Q. of 69 mentally retarded children, ages 5 to 17, whose average I.Q. was 65. For a year they were given 12 grams daily with their food, less than half an ounce.[15] Sure enough, the average gain in the children's I.Q.'s was 11 points, with some rising as much as 17 points. Not only was their problem-solving ability dramatically improved, but so were their personalities. Then, when glutamic acid was no longer given them, they all suffered a sharp decline in I.Q.

In association with Lorene Rogers, Dr. Roger Williams, the noted biochemist who isolated pantothenic acid, raised the I.Q.s of mentally retarded children significantly with another form of glutamic acid, 1-glutamine, which he felt was better metabolized by the brain than glutamic acid.[16]

Dr. Williams recommended 1,100 to 4,000 milligrams daily for adults (both glutamic acid and 1-glutamine can be bought at most health food stores).

Neurotransmitters: Unsung Heroes!

A cliche that's old enough to be retired — too bad it isn't — is, "You are what you eat." It is also inaccurate and incomplete. You are also what you don't eat. There are dietary sins of omission as well as commission. Furthermore, what you eat and don't eat also influences your mind, not just your body.

Until the Wurtman Breakthrough, medical students were told, "Give the brain its quota of glucose and oxygen, and it will make whatever it needs, regardless of the nutrition given the body and your efficiency in metabolizing (burning) nutrients."[17]

This naive belief was shattered by Richard Wurtman and associates at the Massachusetts Institute of Technology who discovered that diet — what you ate for breakfast, lunch or dinner — influences how neurons (nerve cells) in your brain act.

Neurotransmitters, chemical messengers, fire signals from one nerve cell to the other at the speed of lightening. If you are not eating enough of the right foods, the brain can't make these neurotransmitters quickly and efficiently enough for it to function at peak performance.

When rats in the lab of Edith Cohen, a member of the Wurtman team, were fed large amounts of the B vitamin choline, the amounts of the neurotransmitter acetylcholine increased. Later the Wurtmanites found that coline-containing lecithin, a substance derived mainly from egg yolk, milk, soybeans and corn, produced greater amounts of choline in the blood than did choline itself. The high level of choline also lasted much longer than it did when test subjects ate choline itself.[18]

A fascinating discovery of Wurtman and company is that if you eat a meal accenting protein — like, eggs, meat, or fish — you are far more mentally alert than if you eat a meal heavy in carbohydrates, such as fruits or vegetables and cereals. The latter will reduce your thinking efficiency and make you sleepy — not a desirable state in this highly competitive world.

Lecithin: Memory Booster

With a declining ability to remember, one loses the base for building super-intelligence. But good old lecithin helps cope with a bad old memory, as shown by neurologist Barry Baumel, of the Neuromedical Centers of South Florida in Miami, and Florence Safford, social work professor at Florida International University.[19]

If you find yourself going places and losing things — your glasses, keys, your purse or wallet — or you can't recall the right word or you can't remember what's his name, you should consider the Baumel-Safford solution: taking two tablespoons of lecithin granules daily.

Forty 50 to 80 year old volunteers with mild memory loss took this amount of lecithin daily for four weeks. Twenty other test subjects received look-alike placebos. All volunteers kept a log of memory loss incidents for seven days before the experiment and seven days after.

Ninety percent of those on lecithin showed a significant decrease in lapses of memory. However, those on placebos had 60 percent more memory lapses. (Some of the lapses could have been attributed to starting to keep strict score of lapses which hadn't really been done before.)

A big bonus value in 40 percent of the lecithin takers was the upgrading of their emotional condition: They experienced less anxiety and a wonderful state of well-being.

Choline: A Marvel For Mentality

Choline, one of lecithin's main ingredients, is particularly important to mental acuity. It helps to increase the attention span, contributes to the brain's efficiency in taking in information, clarifies thinking and improves memory for recent events.

There are many kinds of neurotransmitters, all dependent on the amount of nutritional raw materials supplied to make them. Over and above these already mentioned basic raw materials for neurotransmitters, there is still another nutrient that influences how quickly and efficiently we learn: the mineral zinc.

Behavioral scientist Mari Golub, at the University of California's primate research center in Davis, studied the use of zinc in 10 rhesus monkeys, a species noted for — you should pardon the expression — aping features of human development and metabolism.[20] Five received only four parts per million of zinc in their daily diet. The other five received 100 parts per million — much more than normal. The zinc-deficient monkeys took two to three times longer than the others to note the difference between a circle and a cross. Further, the zinc-deprived animals had their immune system depressed by 20 to 30 percent.

While the Golub study stated that this degree of zinc-deficiency is unlikely in human beings, it did not seem to recognize that the nation's soils are rapidly becoming zinc-impoverished. In a hearing before the Senate Select Committee on Nutrition and Human Needs, Michael Lesser, M.D. cited government reports which revealed that the soil of 32 states is zinc-deficient and that commercial fertilizers return no zinc to the earth.[21]

How can fruits, vegetables, grains and grasses offer zinc if the soils under them are zinc poor? Can a magician pull a rabbit out of the hat without first having put one in?

Inasmuch as you can't always know where the food you eat was grown or which states are zinc-adequate, it is best to derive zinc from ocean foods, certain select land-grown foods, and/or supplements. (I recommend 25 to 50 milligrams of zinc daily for my patients, according to their needs.)

Although oysters are the richest in zinc, we don't recommend them because oysters — along with crab and clams — are garbage collectors of the sea, often full of harmful pollutants.

Here are other zinc-rich foods and supplements, in number of milligrams per serving of less than four ounces:

herring, 110	torula yeast, 9.9
wheat germ, 14	blackstrap molasses, 8.3
sesame seeds, 10	maple syrup, 7.5

liver, 7.0

soybeans, 6.7

sunflower seeds, 6.6

egg yolk, 5.5

lamb, 5.4

chicken, 4.8

regular molasses, 4.6

brewer's yeast, 3.9

eggs, 2.1

buckwheat, 2.0

oats, 3.7

bone meal, 3.6

rye, 3.4

whole wheat, 3.2

corn, 3.1

coconut and beef, 3.0

beets, turkey and walnuts, 2.8

barley, 2.7

beans and avocados, 22.4

peas, 2.3

bleu cheese, 2.2

How to Exercise Your Brain
and Develop Mental Muscles

In the early 1960s, researchers at the University of California (Berkeley) announced sensational research showing that brain exercise could make the brain larger and more efficient (yet many of us still think that the brain-power we have today is all we'll ever have, so we limit our blast-off to the sky high I.Q).

Professor Marian Diamond, a neuroanatomist, was one of those main researchers in this fascinating field and is now the key researcher there. Her 25 years of experiments with rats have given her rare insight into increasing intelligence in rats and human beings. She says that if we seek challenge and stimulation in our thought lives, we can delay or defeat mental aging and even develop new brain cells, which only a few years ago was believed to be impossible.[22]

Dr. Diamond discovered that there can be brain growth in rats who are 80 to 90 years old in terms of human years. She moved rats who had lived boring lives in uninteresting cages, with only a few companions into, "enriched quarters" — larger cages with many toys and often 12 other rat companions, where the toys were changed daily.

She compared the mental progress of these rats with that of those in the standard, boring cages who had only a few companions. Rats in the enriched environment thrived, socializing and playing with their new toys. The other rats seemed bored, in the same rut, keeping to themselves, hardly moving and acting old.

At the experiment's end, when the rats were more than 120 years old in human terms, those in the enriched environments were found to have increased their number of brain cells. Their cerebral cortex was six percent thicker than that of the bored rats and the topper is that their brains also contained nine percent less lipofuscin, aging pigment.

A Nerve Cell Is A Nerve Cell Is A Nerve Cell

Skeptics say, "This may work for rats, but where is the proof about human beings?" Dr. Diamond says we see it in everyday life: stimulated people stay more mentally acute and active and younger for longer. Besides, she says, clinically, brains are only large clumps of nerve cells, and nerve cells of rats and human beings contain the same basic constituents.

Nerve cells were created to receive stimuli, she continues. They will react positively to stimuli at any age. Brains which meet challenges positively do not lose cells. They gain. We can rev up our I.Q.s by taking a lesson from Brother Rat. We can keep our minds stimulated. We can socialize, we can meet challenging people or ideas in newspapers, magazines and books. We can limber up our brains by exercises, by thinking up solutions to such problems as narcotics, how we would apportion the national budget, or best protect the fast-depleting rain forests of the planet.

Some of my patients exercise their minds by reading titles of fiction books, motion pictures or plays and figuring out the plots. Then they read the book, see the movie or the play to learn how it came out. It doesn't matter if their plot is different, it's the exercise in imagining that counts.

One of my middle-aged patients became so good at this game that she suddenly realized she had unsuspected abilities, and she's now doing something she'd never done before: writing short stories. She sold one recently, now nothing can stop her new career. You think imagining can't help to keep you mentally and physically young — and active, too? Think again.

The choice is yours. You can stay young all your life and enjoy it to the hilt or you can vegetate, isolate yourself, stop using your mind, deteriorate and age rapidly. It doesn't take a psychic to know your choice.

So far as human proof for Dr. Diamond's findings is concerned, you can look to an in-depth study done in the Soviet Union and issued to the United Nations, founded on the tested mental and physical abilities of 21,000 elderly individuals. The conclusion of the Soviet scientists was, "The more that brains and muscles are used, the better they are and the less they age."[23]

A Myth Is As Good As A Mile

Some people program themselves into a downward skid of the I.Q., because, after age 40, they start believing the myth that their brain power declines.

Don't you believe it! Many studies show that the most important forms of intellectual growth can continue into the high 80s.

An incredible number of fine minds start to atrophy because they believe the popular misconception that aging is sure to bring mental deterioration.

This bugs Dr. Warner Schaie of Pennsylvania State University, one of the nation's foremost authorities on aging, who has done many studies that shatter this notion.[24]

"Expecting to decline mentally is a self-fulfilling prophecy," he states. "Those who don't accept the stereotype of a helpless old age, but instead feel they can do as well in old age as they have in other times, don't become ineffective before their time."

Research projects conducted by Schaie and associates over 25 years show that most people retain their intellectual prowess. Imagine, roughly 10 percent of volunteers 74 to 81 years old showed remarkable improvements in test performances of intellectual prowess!

Dr. Jerry Avorn, of the Division on Aging at Harvard Medical School, agrees that we tend to deteriorate, if we tell ourselves we do.[25]

"The deficits found in the healthy aged are in the minor range, not at all clinically impairing. At worst, they're just a nuisance."

Okay then, how do we keep the mental powers we have, or even improve them?

1. Stay socially involved. The I.Q.s of people who become hermits, who are hermetically sealed off from society, pay in deterioration: emotional, physical and mental.

2. Remain mentally active. People who continue to pursue their intellectual curiosities and interests, actually show a dazzling gain in verbal intelligence.

3. Keep your personality flexible. If you get set in your ways, your mind also seems to set and harden like concrete. Is that any way to treat your fine mind?

Individuals who continue enjoying new experiences for a lifetime, have brighter and brighter minds and a far longer and happier lifetime in which to enjoy these new experiences.

Psychologist John Horn of the University of Denver, an authority on intelligence and the aging process, says a group he has studied, the Golden Years Gang, shows its mental youthfulness in being able to look at a subject from many viewpoints. These seniors exhibit their mental alertness and acuity with a rich and fluent way of expressing themselves.[26]

"They can say the same thing in five different ways. In our research, they're better in this sort of knowledge than the young people we see."

Become More Physical
to Become More Mental

About the only physical activity some geniuses get is exercising their imagination. There's much evidence to indicate that they might be super-geniuses if they exercised their body, too.

Over the last generation, numerous studies have pointed out that regular oxygen-using exercises have raised people's problem-solving ability and mental sharpness.

Some years ago the principals at the Perry and Bundy Elementary Schools in Washington, D.C. launched a daily group calisthenics program for the students, lasting one-half hour, from 7:30 to 8:00 AM, when they showered and were provided with breakfast.[27]

The students improved physically and mentally. Intelligence test scores rocketed. Although the benefits were obvious, some critics pooh-poohed the experiment's results because it was more than just daily exercise that influenced the gains. It was also a substantial daily breakfast, which some of the students from poor families hadn't had before.

And this objection was valid. Eaters of a good protein and complex carbohydrate breakfast demonstrated significantly higher intelligence scores than when they had nothing or just a donut and coffee — which is next to nothing.

The low blood sugar level of breakfast-skippers causes more than lower I.Q. scores. Some two-thirds of industrial accidents happen to breakfast-skippers, usually due to poorer manual dexterity.

Within the past few years, a study of the effects of a school breakfast on the conduct and intelligence of elementary school kids showed positive gains. Drs. Alan Meyers and Michael Weitzman of Boston City Hospital, and Amy Sampson of the Tufts School of Nutrition, found less tardiness and absence and an improvement in intelligence scores of the school breakfast eaters — an improvement of almost eight points. Further, the children made fewer mental errors.[28]

Getting The Brain Into Circulation

There's no unfathomable mystery as to why exercise boosts brain-power. It's a matter of enhanced circulation, blood circulation to the brain.

Recently, a researcher at the University of Southern California announced a startlingly higher ability to learn and think while standing on one's feet. Certainly, the act of standing, revs up the metabolism more than just sitting.[29]

Let me (Dr. Langer) tell you of my personal experience. While in medical college, I used to study or memorize as I walked around my room. My roommate would ride me about what he called, "A stupid practice."

Now, the USC study substantiates that I was doing something right, that it wasn't a stupid practice. I get the same results today when I read and pace. I remember much, much better. So, stupid as the practice may seem, it works, and that's pretty close to the bottom line.

So much for improving brain power by stimulating normal circulation with exercise. Much of the adult population — even some youths and children — have arteries that are narrowing with deposits of cholesterol, triglycerides, calcium, fibrin and ceroids and other biochemical gunk. So to get maximum mileage out of the brain, they have to do something to open the arteries for more blood, oxygen and nutrients.

Spring Cleaning For Your Arteries

All right, how can you get back into circulation — the kind that rockets your brain-power out of this world? One way is to make sure your thyroid is working right. (See the earlier reference to the Barnes Basal Temperature Test.)

Several studies indicate that a thyroid in balance can keep the arteries clean — or, in some instances, even clean out some of the blocking debris.

Dr. William B. Kountz studied 288 low thryoid patients with an average age of 67, his patients and others from the infirmary of Washington University, St. Louis, all with high levels of cholesterol and advanced blood disease.[30] Half of the patients received thyroid supplements, the other half, the controls, were given none. After the five year study, Kountz found that the patients on thyroid hormone had only half the fatalities that the controls experienced.

Most alternative doctors find that a daily kelp tablet (available at any health food center) balances the thyroid function in first generation hypothyroids, as stated earlier. However, for second generation hypothyroids and beyond, prescription thyroid such as Armour, natural, desiccated, is needed.

Victory On The High "C"s

A thousand milligrams of vitamin C a day has dramatically lowered cholesterol levels, as demonstrated by Dr. Constance Spittle Leslie, a pathologist at Pinderfields Hospital in Wakefield, Yorkshire, England.

An article by her in Lancet verified the cholesterol-lowering value of 1,000 mg. of vitamin C a day and also stated that it prevented blockages in arteries.[31]

While at Rutgers University some years ago, Dr. Anthony Verlangieri discovered that subnormal intake of vitamin C by rabbits leads to the loss of certain chemical compounds in the artery lining, causing irregularities where harmful plaques begin accumulating. A high intake of vitamin C made these chemicals stay put and assured smooth artery linings.[32]

Folk Remedies To The Rescue

Out of the medicine chest and into the pantry, we find that certain tropical fruits are said to clean out arteries: bananas, kiwi fruit, mangoes and papaya. Certain minerals in them and an enzyme named bromelain supposedly clean out arteries like a pipe cleaner cleans out a pipestem.

Grapefruit and apple pectin are two sleeper items for lowering cholesterol and keeping arteries clean. They are not just folk medicine items. They really work. And there's plenty of solid research underlying these findings.

James Cerda, M.D. of the University of Florida in Gainesville, has conducted many years of research in the pectins — particularly, grapefruit — and has found that 12 grams of grapefruit pectin daily over four months lowered blood cholesterol levels by an average of 17 percent and helped keep the arteries clean of narrowing or blocking biochemical debris.[33] Most surprising, he says this intake of grapefruit pectin can even open narrowing arteries. Good news for your brain and mine!

How many grapefruit a day must a person eat to get the desired results? That's hard to predict, says Cerda. Sometimes you can get 12 grams of pectin daily in just one grapefruit. Other times, it may take six or eight. So those of us shooting for a skyhigh I.Q. would find it much easier to buy tablets or capsules of grapefruit or apple pectin and be assured of the proper number of grams daily.

Most health food stores do not stock grapefruit pectin and don't even know where to buy it. However, since almost all of them carry apple pectin, we asked Dr. Cerda whether apple pectin would work as well and he said, "Yes."[34] So, if you think the pectins will work for you, have at 'em!

Better Circulation With Chelation

Some patients want faster and more decided results in cleaning out their arteries, so they go to chelation, what a Hollywood alternative physician, James Julian, M.D., calls a "roto-rooter" for clogged brain arteries.

A chemical called EDTA is dripped into the bloodstream intravenously and it slowly and safely removes arterial debris, which is passed off through the kidneys. (Added to the EDTA solution are minerals to replace those lost in the chelation process.)

Although orthodox medicine derides chelation, it is both effective and safe. I have sent patients to alternative doctors where chelation treatments are given and have found in almost all cases that they have been helped. EDTA works on all parts of the body and the brain, too.

It is common to see patients — who before were almost senile — once again become aware and reason clearly. Numerous patients have found an amazing return to peak performance mentally — in thinking and remembering — after these treatments.

The Cost Is Reasonable

Generally doctors give chelation in a series of 20 office visits. The cost? In the area of $2,000, more or less. But heart bypasses usually cost 20 or 30 times that much and involve removing arteries from the leg to replace the clogged ones in the heart with.

And, of course, bypass surgery improves circulation only in the heart area, important as that is. Arteries in other parts of the body — and in the brain — remain narrowed or clogged. On the contrary, however, chelation does a thorough housecleaning of arteries throughout the body and brain.

A distressing fact of life is that hardening of the arteries is found increasingly in younger people — now even in small children. Just imagine what this subtle sabotage is doing to the intelligence of America!

There is one hitch to chelation, however. Medicare won't pay for it (although it goes along with expensive bypass surgery), and most insurance companies won't reimburse for chelation treatments either. It doesn't make sense, but when did the government or insurance companies make sense?

Alternative doctors, or labs which give chelation treatment, are in almost all major cities — and some that aren't major. You can find out if one is in your area by word of mouth, through health food stores, or, best of all, through an organization to which most chelating doctors belong: The American College of Advancement in Medicine, 23121 Verdugo Drive, Suite 204, Laguna Hills, CA 92653. The phone number is (714) 583-7666.

The Summing Up

Let's take a quick look at the major principles you've read about in this chapter, to refresh your memory. Then you'll be on your way to going public with the genius within.

First, we mentioned Professor Rivera's system of skyrocketing your I.Q. by 20 to 30 points, then the importance of oxygenating and having normal thyroid function.

Other key considerations are using the Barnes Basal Temperature Test to find out if your thyroid function is low, keeping body temperature up to normal for efficient brain functioning, coping with iron-deficiency anemia, using the vitamins and minerals that are boosters to rocket you into the stratosphere of genius, holding a positive mental attitude and practicing certain brain exercises.

The next stage of rocket boosters to reach the skyhigh I.Q. includes: taking effective physical exercises, eating a nourishing breakfast, and keeping your arteries clear for the free flow of blood, by means of certain nutrients which various studies and folk medicine indicate will clear narrowed arteries, and, through the benefits of chelation, by restoring arteries to a wide-open conditon to carry the most nourishment and oxygen possible to the brain.

That pulls up the zipper on this chapter, signalling the end, but it's a new beginning for you — one that can be a great and richly rewarding adventure — as you apply the principles offered.

There's now a new genius in the making. YOU!

References

1. Personal communication.
2. Nathan Masor, *The New Psychiatry* (New York: Philosophical Library, 1959), 99-100.
3. Ibid.
4. *Complete Book of Vitamins* (Emmaus, PA: Rodale Press, 1976), 507.
5. Louis Berman, *The Glands Regulating Personality* (New York, NY: The Macmillan Company, 1921), 55.
6. Stephen E. Langer with James F. Scheer, *Solved: The Riddle of Illness* (New Canaan, CT: Keats Publishing, Inc., 1984), 4.
7. Noel K. Marshall, "A Chilling Effect," *Psychology Today* (February, 1982): 92.
8. Ibid.
9. Roger J. Williams, *Nutrition Against Disease* (New York, NY: Pitman Publishing Corporation, 1971): 65.
10. Ibid.
11. *The Health Finder* (Emmaus, PA: Rodale Books, Inc., 1954), 839-40.
12. Ibid., 839.
13. Ibid.
14. Jeffrey Bland, *Nutraerobics* (San Francisco, CA: Harper and Row Publishers, 1983), 315-316.
15. Catharyn Elwood, *Feel Like A Million* (New York, NY: Pocket Books, 1968), 258.
16. Roger J. Williams, *Nutrition Against Disease* (New York, NY: Pitman Publishing Corporation, 1971), 164.

17. *Science*, Vol 203, January 5, 1979, 36.

18. Ibid.

19. "Lecithin Makes Memory Function," *San Francisco Chronicle*, April 3, 1983, B-7.

20. *Science News*, Vol 134, No. 2, July 9, 1988, 27.

21. Stephen E. Langer with James F. Scheer, *Solved, The Riddle of Weight Loss* (Rochester, Vermont: Healing Arts Press, 1989), 166.

22. Stephen E. Langer with James F. Scheer, *Solved: The Riddle of Illness* (New Canaan, CT: Keats Publishing, Inc., 1984), 138-139.

23. Ibid.

24. "Intelligence Can Rise as Folks Enter Old Age," Register (Orange County, CA), April 12, 1984, E-9.

25. Ibid.

26. Ibid.

27. *Science Newsletter*, 84:9, July 6, 1963.

28. *Bestways*, April, 1985, 16.

29. Ibid., April, 1989, 19.

30. Stephen E. Langer with James F. Scheer, *Solved: The Riddle of Illness* (New Canaan, CT: Keats Publishing, Inc., 1984), 109-110.

31. Ibid., 111.

32. Ibid., 110.

33. Jean Carper, *The Food Pharmacy* (New York, NY: Bantam Books, 1987), 322.

34. Personal communication.

Flushes Fat
Right Out
Of
Your Arteries

Dr. William H. Lee

Preventive Medicine Instead of a Coronary Bypass

You can change your life-style and . . . without drugs or surgery, halt or reverse atherosclerosis, the artery-hardening disease that can lead to a heart attack.

Who said that?

Some quack wanting to peddle snake oil while getting rich in the process?

No! It was said by Doctor Alexander Leaf, Director of the Cardiovascular Health Center at Massachusetts General Hospital in Boston . . . and it shook up a lot of physician's thinking about the treatment of heart disease.

As quoted in the New York Times, November 15, 1988, Dr. Leaf said, "It's extremely important to show that without drugs, just by changing people's life-style, you can get coronary artery disease to regress."

A research team led by Dr. Dean Ornish, an assistant clinical professor of medicine at the University of California - San Francisco, said, "If the results continue to be as good from the study, it will be very important in making physicians consider alternatives to heart transplants, bypasses and other high tech medicines."

The subjects of the study which revealed this information had all been told, on the basis of an angiogram, that they had severe heart disease. Fifty patients were randomly divided into two groups. One group received traditional care including advice on lowering their cholesterol levels and blood pressure as well as advice on quitting smoking.

The second group were put on a low-fat vegetarian diet with about 10% of calories to be obtained from fat, plus an exercise program, stress-management training and no smoking.

The second group had a measurable widening of arteries. The greatest improvement came in the arteries that had been the most clogged!

Cholesterol in the blood is a primary cause of the progressive blocking. In the treatment group, total cholesterol averaged 213 milligrams per deciliter of blood before beginning. After life-style change, a year later it averaged 154.

The study will help to change the attitudes of cardiologists if it continues to show that coronary heart disease *can* melt away. Dr. Leaf said, "Now more cardiologists may be willing to do some preventive medicine instead of waiting to do a coronary bypass."

Studies continue and many substances other than prescription drugs can help you to lower your serum cholesterol . . . and they won't cost you an arm and a leg either. For example, a report published in the *Journal of The American Medical Association*, found that the amount of oat bran needed to lower cholesterol by 13% in a year (1 1/2 cups daily) would cost $249.00. A year's worth of the prescription drug *cholestyramine* — which is the amount needed to gain the same result — would cost $1,442.00, and the drug *colestipol* would cost $879.00.

Some substances are exotic (Hershouwu, a traditional Chinese medication), or strange (fish-oil fed chickens), lemongrass oil or Japanese green tea. Others, just as powerful or even more powerful are available at your neighborhood health food store.

When it comes to coronary combat, there's more ammunition at your disposal than you ever thought!

Cholesterol

Cholesterol is a white, waxy substance that is classified as a fat.

Although it is usually thought of as being in the bloodstream, and that fact has received the most publicity, it is actually a part of all tissues.

Cholesterol is essential to life.

It is part of the structure of the cell's outer membrane.

It provides an insulation shield around nerve fibers.

It serves as a building block for the manufacture of certain hormones in the body.

Cholesterol is so important that the body manufactures it in the liver.

So, some cholesterol is not dangerous . . . *however, too much cholesterol in certain parts of the body can be deadly!*

Cholesterol and other fats can build up in the bloodstream and accumulate on the walls of the blood vessels until the accumulation impairs the circulation. If the accumulation continues until the circulation is cut off, it can lead to a heart attack or a stroke.

The liver manufactures about 1,000 milligrams of cholesterol a day. In addition, our diet provides another 500 milligrams or more. Cholesterol is a part of the animal products we consume. Products such as meat, eggs, fish, poultry, and dairy products.

Although not gospel, the cholesterol equation appears to go this way:

The liver combines proteins, fats (triglycerides) and cholesterol into mixture. The mixture is called very-low-density-lipoproteins (VLDL). As the VLDL mixture circulates throughout the body, it drops off the triglycerides to muscle cells to be used for energy or to fat cells for storage.

When VLDL drops off the triglycerides it becomes low-density-lipoprotein (LDL).

The LDL then carries the cholesterol through the system dropping it off in the areas that need it for cell building, and dumping the balance into the bloodstream.

That's one mixture the liver makes.

The liver makes another combination called high-density-lipoprotein (HDL). It is also made up of protein, choelsterol and fat, but, in this mixture, the fat is a phospholipid. HDL also contains less cholesterol. As the HDL circulates through the bloodstream it picks up the floating cholesterol it comes in contact with and brings it back to the liver for reprocessing or excretion.

Therefore, the LDL has been termed "bad" cholesterol and the HDL is called "good" cholesterol.

LDL is made up primarily of saturated fats (generally fats which are solid at room temperature - butter, bacon fat, meat fats, coconut and palm oil).

HDL is made up primarily of fats which are liquid at room temperature (corn, safflower, sesame, soybean oils, etc.).

Therefore, it appears that a dietary intake of saturated fat will raise the serum cholesterol content while dietary intake of unsaturated or monosaturated oils (olive oil) will either not raise the serum cholesterol level or, in some cases, lower it.

Suggested Optimum Cholesterol Levels

Age	Males Total	LDL	Females Total	LDL
Under 20	150	90	160	90
20 - 40	190	110	195	110
40 - 60	200	120	210	120
Over 60	210	140	210	140

It is important for you to bring your cholesterol levels to these numbers approximately, noting that there is a ratio between total cholesterol and LDL cholesterol.

A number of factors affect the total cholesterol level in the bloodstream, many of which you can help control:

* Exercise
* Alcohol consumption
* Smoking
* Obesity
* Saturated Fat consumption
* Unsaturated Fat consumption
* Fish, Fiber consumption
* Consumption of foods high in preformed cholesterol (eggs, meat, whole milk, etc.)

There are also other nutritional factors which lend you a hand in controlling cholesterol. They include the vitamin niacin, EPA, garlic, lecithin, phosphatidyl choline, GLA, onions, L-carnitine, Coenzyme Q-10 and so on.

These are nature's gifts which we only have to know about in order to use. Many have been tested in double-blind studies while some have been used by herbalists through the centuries because they work. They will be presented to you in no particular order and with no preference because we are all individuals and, although all of them work, some may work better for you than others.

When you decide to try one or more of them, remember that they are not drugs. We are accustomed to taking a tablet like an aspirin and expect immediate relief. These are natural substances and the body needs time to work them into the system for the most benefit. Six to twelve weeks is a good trial period. Don't be impatient. It's worth the effort.

Lemongrass Oil Can
Lower Your Cholesterol

Departments of Nutritional Sciences and Medicine, University of Wisconsin.

A vegetarian diet has been shown to be protective to the heart. Some of the protection afforded comes from mevalonate metabolites found in lemongrass oil.

When tested for 90 days on high-cholesterol males, 36% responded to the oil with more than a 10% decrease in serum cholesterol. The diet they ate was not changed so the reduction had to come from the supplement.

Chickens Fed Fish Oil
Produce Lower Cholesterol Food

You may be able to eat eggs without worrying about their effect on your heart if the diet of the laying hens has been enriched with omega 3 fatty acids (found in fish oil).

The University of Utah and Utah State University have been conducting experiments to increase the omega 3 content of eggs. Eggs from the laying hens fed diets supplemented with Max Epa (fish oil) were found to have increased omega 3 value and decreased cholesterol content.

When tests were run with subjects eating regular eggs, there was an increase in plasma levels of cholesterol and triglycerides as expected. However, when omega 3 enriched eggs were consumed, cholesterol levels remained unchanged and triglyceride levels decreased.

Don't run to the supermarket for these eggs yet. As you may have suspected, they do taste a bit like fish. A little more work has to be done before they are acceptable to the American taste . . .

Coffee, Tea and Coronary Disease

New England Journal of Medicine, Oct. 16, 1977

Investigators at Johns Hopkins reported on the experiences of 1,000 white male physicians who have been studied for an average of 25 years on coffee consumption. Subjects who drank 3 to 4 cups a day had about twice as many coronary events as those who drank none. Those who drank about 5 cups a day had 2.8 times as many coronary events.

However, opinion is still divided about coffee's role in coronary disease since heavy coffee drinkers are usually heavy smokers as well.

Tea tannins, on the other hand, are found to lower cholesterol. The catechins (tannins) in green tea lower cholesterol levels and may have a protective effect against the atherosclerotic process. According to a study by K. Muramatsu, M. Fukuyo and Y. Hara in the *Journal of Nutrition Science and Vitaminology,* Vol. 32, 1986, tests were conducted with cholesterol-fed rats, and then on humans who habitually drank tea with a high cholesterol diet (3 eggs per meal).

Despite the fact that they were eating a high cholesterol diet, those who drank green tea had cholesterol levels within the normal range.

Understanding Oil Labels

If the label reads	The product may contain
partially hydrogenated vegetable shortening	coconut, soybean, or corn
hydrogenated vegetable shortening	soybean, palm, or palm kernel
100% vegetable oil	palm, palm kernel, cotton-seed, peanut, soybean, olive, canola, sunflower, safflower

Why is it important to know the kind of oil you are getting?

According to *Environmental Nutrition*, Vol. 11, No. 1, pp. 1.3, saturated tropical oils such as palm, palm kernel, and palm oil, which are commonly used in processed foods, may *even be more saturated than animal fats*, raise blood cholesterol levels and increase a person's risk of heart disease.

Manufacturers often replace soybean oil, which is low in saturated fat, with the cheaper but more saturated palm oils. Yet, to you, cost is not the only issue. Tropical oils (palm, palm kernel, coconut) may have an impact on heart disease. This is especially important when they replace unsaturated and monosaturated oils like canola, olive, sesame, peanut, soybean, safflower, and sunflower. These oils do not have the same adverse effect on the heart.

NOTE: It's a good idea to use vitamin E supplements any time you use oils in the diet. Vitamin E helps to protect the oils from rancidity.

You can determine which oils are in your food by reading the labels and deciphering what they really mean.

Fake Fats, Safe or Unsafe?

Want to gorge yourself on french fries cooked in fat that has no calories? Satisfy your craving for that greasy taste without raising your cholesterol level? Maybe the answer is Olestra from Procter & Gamble.

Olestra is made from natural sugar and vegetable oil bonded together into a molecule that's too large to be digested or absorbed by the body so it's calorie and cholesterol free any may also actually inhibit the absorption of cholesterol from other foods.

Too good to be true?

Maybe so. It was in 1987 that Procter & Gamble petitioned the FDA for approval to market Olestra. According to *Nutrition Report* July, 1988, Mr. Melvin Reuber, in a report submitted by the Center for Science in the Public Interest to the FDA, Olestra may be a harmful substance.

So when you're reading labels, you might want to avoid fake fats until there's a real clean bill of health. Also, consider the fact that even though we've had artificial sweeteners on the market for years with loads of people consuming fake sugars, people in the United States eating the good old American diet are as obese and prone to cardiac problems as ever . . .

Dr. Kenneth H. Cooper, M.D., America's aerobic guru has written about three vices and their impact on cholesterol. You guessed it. Drinking coffee, alcohol and smoking raise havoc with your cholesterol level. But other factors also enter into the cholesterol equation. The stress connection (and who isn't stressed . . . emotional stress — occupational problems — job loss — surgery, etc.) can knock your cholesterol values out of whack. Too much anxiety and pressure in your life can have a negative and even dangerous impact on your psychological and physiological well-being.

How Can You Combat Stress?

1) Start an aerobic exercise program. You'll soon find that the movements trigger the release of natural tranquilizers in the brain called endorphins.
2) Practice relaxation techniques (buy a good book such as the *Relaxation Response* by Herbert Benson, M.D. (Morrow Press, 1975).
3) Get involved in supportive relationships.
4) Reduce your stress level by rearranging your daily schedule to include free time.

Your Age Makes a Difference

Cholesterol levels increase with age. More so for women than men as far as the HDL (high density level cholesterol) is concerned, but the total cholesterol and the LDL (low-density level cholesterol) increase for both sexes at a faster rate. Possibly because you are eating the same as you always did but burning off less fat. Cut your caloric intake and exercise more.

What's Your Number?

When you get your cholesterol level checked, you will see numbers, acronyms, ratios, total values, etc. What do they all mean? What should your "numbers" be?

Total Cholesterol:

In the mid-1950s the "safe" range was thought to be 150 to 350 milligrams per deciliter (mg/dl). How thinking has changed during the intervening 30 years!

Recommendation:

186-209 mg/dl for both sexes, age 40-59.
189-213 for males 60-plus.
205-227 for females 60-plus.

LDLs (Low-Density Lipoproteins):

These are the main carriers of cholesterol in the blood - the so-called "bad" cholesterol. The higher this level is, the more trouble you're in.

Recommendation:

119-140 for males 40-59.
110-128 for females 40-59.
122-143 for males 60-plus.
126-149 for females 60-plus.

HDLs (High-Density Lipoproteins):

These transport cholesterol from the body's tissues to the liver, where cholesterol is eliminated; hence the term "good" cholesterol.

Recommendation:

More than 52 for males 40-59.
More than 69 for females 40-59.
More than 60 for males 60-plus.
More than 74 for females 60-plus.

Total Cholesterol to HDL Cholesterol Ratio:

The higher your ratio is, the greater your risk of having a cardiovascular problem, so the lower the better.

Recommendation:

2.6-4.2 for males 40-59.
2.0-3.0 for females 40-59.
2.5-4.0 for males 60-plus.
2.0-3.2 for females 60-plus.

Triglycerides:

These are not cholesterol but fatty molecules in your blood. A growing body of thought implicates triglycerides in the destructive process of altherosclerosis.

Recommendation:

89-121 for males 40-59.
73-98 for females 40-59.
83-110 for males 60-plus.
82-110 for females 60-plus.

Oats For Your Arteries

Eating a bowl of oat bran along with a stack of pancakes covered with butter and syrup will not help your cholesterol balance. You will have to look for ways to reduce the amount of fat in your breakfast as well as other meals. If you don't want to make your own oatmeal, there are a number of ready-made products that can help you to add oat bran to your regular diet.

Some products are better for you than others. Read labels to find whether or not the contents promise more than they can deliver.

American Journal of Clinical Nutrition 34(5):824-9, 1981
Experimental controlled study — Oat-bran intake selectively lowers serum low-density lipoprotein, cholesterol concentrations of hypercholesterolemic men. (Kirby RW et al.)

Control and oat-bran diets were given in alternating sequence to a group of men exhibiting high cholesterol. Their diet was not changed other than the inclusion of the oat-bran.

Total cholesterol was reduced 13%, plasma LDL cholesterol was lowered 14% and the HDL cholesterol was unchanged.

Some Examples of Experimental Studies
For Those Who Want to Investigate Further

Guar Gum
Subjects used five grams of guar gum daily for 12 weeks. Total cholesterol decreased 13.8%.
(*Nutr. Rep. Int.* 31(3):505-20, 1985)

Grapefruit Pectin
Lowered serum and tissue cholesterol levels.
(*American Journal of Clinical Nutrition* 34:50-53, 1981)

Niacin
Should be the first substance to be used when diet fails to adequately reduce LDL cholesterol levels.
(*Journal of the American Medical Association* 255 (4):512-21, 1986)

Vitamin C
At a rate of 3 grams daily, 79 males showed a significant decrease in cholesterol after three weeks.
(*Aliment. Nutr. Metab.* 2(3): 169-182, 1981)

Calcium
Total serum cholesterol decreased significantly with 1,025 to 1,200 milligrams of calcium.
(*Nutrition Reports Int.*, August 1973)

PRODUCT	DIETARY FIBER (g)	COMMENT
BREAKFAST CEREALS (1 OZ.)		
Oat Bran (Quaker)	4	Pure oat bran. Hot cereal; can be used in baking.
Oat Bran (Erewhon)	3	Contains oat bran and wheat germ.
Oats, Old-fashioned or Quick (Quaker)	2.7	Oats only, no additives. Can be ground into oat flour in blender.
Oatmeal, Instant (Quaker)	2	Flavored varieties contain added fat and sugar. High in sodium.
Oatmeal, Instant (Arrowhead Mills)	4	Oats only.
Oatmeal, 30-second (Maypo)	2	Made from whole-grain oat flour. Fortified with vitamins and minerals.
Cheerios (General Mills)	2	Made from whole-grain oat flour. Fortified with vitamins and minerals.
Oat Bran O's (Health Valley)	2.8	Cold cereal containing fruit juices and other grains besides oats and oat bran.
Cracklin' Oat Bran (Kellogg)	5	Cold cereal containing oat bran, wheat bran, three kinds of sugar, coconut, and coconut oil. High in saturated fat.
BREAD (1 slice)		
Oatmeal Bread, 1.5-lb. loaf (Pepperidge Farm)	1.5	Chiefly white (wheat) flour, plus some oatmeal.
Five Star Fibre, Harvest Wheat (Pepperidge Farm)	2.5	Chiefly white (wheat) flour, plus oats and other grains.
CRACKERS (1 oz.)		
7 Grain Vegetable, Stoned (Health Valley)	2.75	Chiefly whole-wheat Wheat flour, amaranth, barley malt, and oats. Fairly high in poly-unsaturated fat (safflower oil).
Oat Bran Graham (Health Valley)	3	Chiefly whole-wheat flour, oat bran, soy oil, and fruit juice.

Harvard Medical School Newsletter, October, 1988

Chromium
 Decreased LDL and increased HDL were observed after 12 weeks
 on 200 micrograms of chromium daily.
 (*American Journal of Clinical Nutrition* 34:2670-8, 1981)

Carnitine
 Improved free fatty acid metabolism.
 (*Int. J. Cardiol.* 5:213, 1984)

Phytosterols
 May decrease cholesterol absorption, even in the absence of
 dietary cholesterol.
 (*Canadian Journal of Biochemistry and Physiology* 36:895, 1958)

Coenzyme-Q
 Improved exercise tolerance.
 (*Biomedical and Clinical Aspects of Coenzyme-Q*, Vol. 2, 1980)

Omega-3 Fatty Acids
 Fish oil diet led to marked decreases in total cholesterol,
 triglycerides and VLD cholesterol.
 (*New England Journal of Medicine* 312:1210-6, 1985)

Phosphatidyl Choline
 Supplementation may not only improve lipoprotein metabolism but
 may cause regression of plaques.
 (*Brit. J. Exp. Path.* 66:35-46, 1985)

Alfalfa
 Rich in saponins which are capable of binding to cholesterol and
 bile salts in the gut to prevent absorption.
 (*American Journal of Clinical Nutrition* 1810-12, 1979)

Garlic & Onion
   Supplementation may protect against atherogenesis.
   (*Atherosclerosis* 26:379-82, 1977)

Ginkgo Biloba
   Supplementation may protect against arterial hypoxia.
   (*Arzneim-Forsch* 35:1283-6, 1985)

Activated Charcoal
   Supplementation may reduce triglycerides and may reduce LDL
   while raising HDL cholesterol.
   (*Lancet*, 2:366-67, 1986)

Harvard Medical School Health Letter, September 1987.
   "Cholesterol: Pills and Powders"
   " . . . niacin is now rather widely used to lower cholesterol
   because it is quite effective as well as relatively safe and
   inexpensive."

Parade Magazine February 22, 1987, Page 8.
   "Should You Take Vitamins?" Dr. Stuart Berger
   "A 1975 study in the Journal of the American Medical
   Association reported that heart patients taking niacin reduced post-
   heart attack risk by 29 percent. And a key study in the New
   England Journal of Medicine found that niacin seems to boost the
   action of certain cholesterol-lowering drugs by up to 25 percent
   and may actually help reverse atherosclerosis."

Vitamin Information Medical Update Hoffman-LaRoche
   "Potential for Nicotinic Acid as Prophylactic Against Coronary
   Heart Disease"
   "Nicotinic acid or its precursor beta-pyridylcarbinol can significantly reduce the plasma levels of low-density lipoproteins (LDL)
   and triglycerides, the fats which are considered to predispose
   towards atherosclerosis, and raise high-density lipoproteins (HDL),
   which are thought to protect against atherosclerosis."

The Wall Street Journal, October 5, 1987.
"Doctor's Orders: Cholesterol Study Calls for Broad Treatment Change"
"They (government sponsored panel) also recommended as a first-line of treatment, nicotinic acid, which is also the vitamin niacin."

The New York Times, October 5, 1987.
"U.S. Defines Cholesterol Hazards and Offers Treatment Guidelines."
"If six months of dieting fails, the guidelines recommend that drugs be considered in addition to continuation of the diet. The drugs 'of first choice' are considered the bile sequesterants, such as cholestyramine and colestipol, and nicotinic acid whose long-term safety and effect in reducing the risk of heart disease have been established."

The New York Times, June 19, 1987.
"For First Time, Cut in Cholesterol is Shown to Deter Artery Clogging"
"Half the men were given daily doses of two drugs, colestipol and niacin, and were put on a diet that was low in fat, calories, and cholesterol."
"The study showed that 16.2 percent of those on the drug and diet treatment experienced dramatic shrinkage of fat deposits all over their bodies, as against only 2.4 percent of those taking placebos."

Mens' Health, September, 1985.
"Niacin Reduces Post-Heart Attack Risk"
"Sixteen years after 1,119 male heart attack survivors began taking niacin, a B-vitamin, the group had an 11 percent lower death rate than a similar group of men given a placebo (sugar pill), investigators found."
"Niacin, which protects against atherosclerosis by lowering blood lipids (cholesterol and triglycerides), was one of five lipid-lowering agents tested on over 8,000 male heart attack survivors in the Coronary Drug Project. Niacin was found to be the most

effective of the five agents which included clofibrate, dextroth-
yroxine and two types of estrogen, or female sex hormones."

Science and Technology, Business Week, December 23, 1985.
"A Home Remedy That's Good for Your Heart"
"In a two year study of 72 patients, niacin lowered the cholesterol
level an average of 11%. For those who took the maximum
dosage of 1000 mg, cholesterol fell 37%."

U.S. News and World Report, June 29, 1987.
"Results of Latest Study, Killer Cholesterol: The News is Good"
"About half were put on a cholesterol-lowering diet and given two
cholesterol-lowering agents, colestipol and niacin. The cholesterol
levels in these men dropped by 26 percent in two years, while in
the untreated men, the drop was only 4 percent,"

T & G-2 F-D-C Reports, June 22, 1987.
"Upjohn's Colestid Caused Plaque Regression in 16% of Patients"
"The colestipol-niacin therapy also produced a major reduction in
total plasma cholesterol (26%) compared to a relative small
decrease for placebo subjects (4%). Similar differences between
the two study groups were observed for LDL cholesterol (43%
vs. 5% reduction) and triglycerides (22% vs 5% reduction). Blood
concentration of HDL cholesterol increased 37% in the treatment
group but only 2% in the placebo subjects."

L-Carnitine, Burns Fat From Within

Although not considered to be an essential nutrient because it
can be manufactured in the body, carnitine plays an important role in
converting fat into energy. It transfers fatty acids to the cell's engine
which uses them as an energy source.

Carnitine is biosynthesized in the liver and is found in the
highest concentrations in skeletal muscle, heart muscle and organs. In
the human diet, it is those meats which supply carnitine for body use.

Carnitine can be manufactured from the amino acids lysine and
methionine but not in adequate levels for all human beings.

Vegetarians are more susceptible to deficiencies in these amino acids. Also, in order for carnitine to be manufactured, sufficient amounts of vitamin B-3, B-6, C and the mineral iron must be present at the same time.

As a fat converter, L-carnitine has been found beneficial for cardiovascular patients and athletes. It assists in regulating fat metabolism in heart and skeletal muscles. Some of its cardiovascular benefits includes reduction of blood triglycerides and cholesterol.

A lack of L-carnitine can result in obesity because of a fat build-up. Daily supplementation will definitely improve the situation. Supplementation is also beneficial to the athlete because it produces efficient fat burning necessary during prolonged physical exercise. It is even more important because the level of fat burned thus rises to as much as 60 percent during the exercise period.

In the absence of L-carnitine, many fats cannot be burned and therefore build up within the cell and the bloodstream as fats and triglycerides. It also plays an important role in the production of heat in "brown fat." Brown fat is the fat tissue that helps us acclimate to cold temperatures and is thought to help determine how much of the food we eat is burned for heat and how much is converted into stored body-fat.

The major sources of dietary carnitine are meat and dairy products. Vegetables, fruits and cereals contain little or no L-carnintine.

Supplements are available in 250 milligrams doses or in complex formulas. Follow label directions.

Phytosterols,
A Natural Approach to Cholesterol Control

Although, as we have said before, cholesterol is essential to normal well-being in appropriate amounts, excess cholesterol from foods can be dangerous. Twenty to thirty percent of the circulating cholesterol comes from our diet. In 1984, the National Heart, Lung, and Blood Institute (NHLBI) studied the relationship between cholesterol and heart disease. They concluded that the *investigation of over 3,800 male subjects showed that the risk of heart attack deaths dropped 2 percent for every one percent reduction in serum cholesterol.*

So, who are we kidding?

The decrease in the intake of cholesterol could save your life.

If you won't cooperate by changing your diet, by exercising . . . at least use some of the helpers nature has put on this earth.

The dietary guidelines include:

* no more than 30% of diet calories from fat
* no more than 10% from saturated fat
* reduce your cholesterol intake to 250 to 300 milligrams daily.

Grains, nuts, fruits and vegetables are cholesterol-free but also make a boring diet to most of us. We like eggs, meat and dairy products. The next best thing is to cut down on the intake and use something like the phytosterols.

What Are They?

Chemically, phytosterols resemble cholesterol in structure. They are found in the more helpful foods like grains, seeds, nuts and fruit. The three phytosterols which have shown the greatest value are called *beta-sitosterol, stigmasterol,* and *campesterol.*

Not your everyday names but you'll see why it pays to know them. The first real demonstration of reduced serum cholesterol levels was done by a Doctor O. J. Pollack way back in 1952. Since then there have been over 100 studies involving nearly 2,000 human beings. In the vast majority of the cases (remember that we are all individuals so what works well for some people may not work as well for all of the people), the result was a *significant reduction in cholesterol levels. Taking phytosterols with a meal decreased cholesterol absorption by as much as 64%.*

The majority of the evidence gathered from animal and human studies suggest that phytosterols appear to slow the absorption of dietary cholesterol and increase its excretion. In addition, they may not only improve your body's ability to burn fat, but also wash away deadly plaques in your arteries.

How Does It Work?

The exact blocking mechanism is still not known. Some theories include:

* the formation of a non-absorbable complex in the intestine
* inhibition of cholesterol uptake at the site of absorption
* reduction of the solubility of cholesterol

However, there's more to the phytosterol story. Because phytosterols also reduce serum cholesterol even if there is no intake of dietary cholesterol, it is suggested that they may inhibit the reabsorption of a portion of the recirculating cholesterol that is a normal constituent of the bile in the intestine.

How Much Is Needed?

A daily intake of 300 milligrams of phytosterols, based on beta-sitosterol content, has been shown to have a significant effect on lowering serum cholesterol. This would be approximately 100 milligrams to be taken as a dietary supplement at each meal.

Oats Against Cholesterol: A Delicious Weapon

Dietary fiber is part of the plant food that is not digested in the small intestine. The fiber receiving the most publicity has been wheat bran, the "bran" in most cereals. Wheat bran's ability to improve regularity is well known and is due to components (lignin, cellulose and hemicellulose) that are not soluble in water.

The insoluble fiber is the material that has the ability to speed fecal transit time and promote bowel health.

Soluble fiber, however, has little effect on regularity. On the other hand, soluble fiber has been shown to lower cholesterol in humans and animals.

In an experiment, men with serum cholesterol (250/dl) added 50 grams of oatmeal to their daily diet (4.5 grams a day). The results were slow but definite. After 8 weeks there was an average drop of six percent in the serum cholesterol level.

The fiber skyrockets the rate your body breaks down and pounds out cholesterol. It may also bind some of the bile acids fording the HDL to transport more cholesterol from the blood to be converted to bile acid. When more HDL is needed, less LDL is produced by the liver.

Oat bran is easily enjoyed in muffins but if you don't like oat bran as a food you can find it in a tablet at your health food store.

Lemongrass Oil

Vegetarians appear to have less problems with cholesterol and corresponding vascular difficulties. Scientists at the Departments of Nutritional Science and Medicine, University of Wisconsin have come to the conclusion that the vegetable protection is afforded by substances called mevalonate metabolites.

They are in adequate amounts in lemongrass oil, so the researchers used it to explore their hypothesis. Males with higher than normal amounts of serum cholesterol were given 140 milligrams of lemongrass oil daily for three months. Thirty-six percent of the volunteers in the test showed a decrease better than ten percent of serum cholesterol. The test group did not change their diet.

This is a preliminary test and more work is needed before the ultimate value of lemongrass oil is determined.

From China with Some Doubt

The value of traditional Chinese herbal medicine is really not appreciated in the United States. In spite of a 5,000 year tradition, most medical authorities discount the effects of herbal medicine. In this case, however, scientists at Oklahome State University teamed up with the U.S. Department of Agriculture to test a herb called *hershouwu*.

An extract of hershouwu was given to four groups of laboratory animals. The results were that serum cholesterol concentrations were significantly reduced.

In this case, when the traditional herb was tested it performed exactly as expected. However, unless it is sold as a dietary supplement without any claims, don't expect to find it on store shelves.

Activated Charcoal

This is not the charcoal you use in your grill. It's a different form of charcoal prepared from wood, nutshells or vegetable matter roasted *without oxygen* to a glossy black. It is then ground into very fine particles and steamed at very high temperatures to open the pinpoint pores which dot each particle's surface.

These pores have the ability to latch on to certain fluids and gases. This ability makes activated charcoal a natural, all-purpose filter. It's in pads for sneakers to control odors but it's also used in a purified form to counteract poisons when people have accidentally swallowed something they shouldn't have. It also counteracts drug overdoses and has been used to relieve people with stomach gas problems.

Activated charcoal is quite an active agent and it now is being put to use when there is excess serum cholesterol. Early results suggest taking activated charcoal may be more effective than some of the conventional drug treatments.

Seven patients in Finland were given about a quarter-ounce of activated charcoal three times a day for four weeks. Even in that short a time, the level of cholesterol (LDL) fell 43 percent. At the same time, levels of HDL rose slightly.

It appears that activated charcoal coming in contact with cholesterol binds to it and removes it from the body along with the waste material. It simply picks up the cholesterol and safely moves it out of the body.

Is there a negative side to activated charcoal? You have to take capsules because it is a little bit gritty and it may cause a bit of constipation. But, that's a small price to pay.

Glucomannan (Amorphophallus Konjac)

Konjac mannan is a polysaccharide derived from the tubers of the konjac tree. It was first introduced as an appetite supressant in 1982. It has been used for hundreds of years in Japan and is a distant relative of the yam. Commonly found in health food stores in tablet or capsule form under the name glucomannan, it was promoted as a weight-aid because it is a rich, non-nutritive fiber that is able to expand to about 50 times its mass but is not absorbed or utilized by the body. It is believed to work by surrounding foods with the increased mass. Therefore it speeds killer food through your body, allowing less time to absorb fats and sugars.

According to the J. Nutrition 97:382, glucomannan has been shown to reduce plasma cholesterol levels in rats. Rats fed high cholesterol diets containing 3% glucomannan for 7 days exhibited 16 percent lower plasma cholesterol levels than rats fed an identical diet without the glucomannan.

At high doses of purified glucomannan, rats had 23 percent lower cholesterol levels than control groups. It is possible that the dual effect of weight control and lower serum cholesterol may bring glucomannan into more prominence in the future as additional laboratory experiments confirm its ability. In other words, it not only lowers cholesterol, but controls ugly fat.

Guar Gum

Guar gum is a natural product similar in action to glucomannan. It is a gelatin-like fiber which combines with the fluids in the stomach and intestines to increase bulk.

Guar gum comes from a plant that has been grown for centuries in Pakistan and India and is now grown in the United States. When guar gum is taken before meals it makes you eat far less because of the balloon feeling in your stomach. The use of about 15 grams a day helps reduce body weight and cholesterol.

The possible negative effect of guar gum and glucomannan is that by hurrying food through the gastrointestinal tract or by shielding food from digestive juices, the body may lack certain important nutrients. Therefore, it is essential that people using these products eat at least one meal a day, without the use of guar gum or glucomannan, that is diet-balanced for health. Or, make sure that enough supplements are taken to prevent possible deficiencies.

Niacin — The Vitamin That Lowers Cholesterol

Increased intake of niacin (vitamin B-3) has been shown to lower the mortality rate of men who have suffered previous heart attacks. This inexpensive vitamin can reduce the risk of heart disease far better than diet alone, a placebo, or any of five commonly prescribed drugs. (*Healthfacts*, May 1986, Arthur A. Levin, M.P.H.)

Researchers at the University of Cincinnati Medical Center investigated the cholesterol-lowering effects of therapies including varying combinations of Lovastatin, resin, and niacin.

The combination of the three lowered total cholesterol 48 percent, LDL cholesterol 59 percent and the ratio of LDL to HDL cholesterol 65 percent. HDL cholesterol was raised 20 percent. (*Arteriosclerosis* 1987; 7:517 A)

The combination of Colestipol and niacin is an effective treatment for atherosclerosis, say state researchers at the University of Southern California.

The combination of the two agents reduced total plasma cholesterol 26 percent, LDL cholesterol 43 percent, and plasma triglycerides 22 percent. HDL cholesterol (the good cholesterol) was increased by 37 percent. (*Arteriosclerosis* 1987; 7:508 A)

Niacin can be very helpful to you if you have to reduce your serum cholesterol. There is one drawback to using this vitamin and that is the niacin flush. It is the result of histamine release and vasodilation, not dangerous, but alarming if you do not expect it to happen. It usually occurs on the face, head, neck, arms and chest. The face looks flushed and the skin feels warm. In some cases even a little itchy. It lasts up to 3/4 of an hour and then subsides without any ill effects. Some people even get to like the feeling after a time.

You can keep the flush to a minimum by beginning your niacin program with 50 milligrams three times a day and gradually building the strength. Or, you can take your niacin with meals to see if that does the trick.

Perhaps the best way is to take 500 or 600 milligrams of niacin in a timed-release form. This is a special form of niacin which gradually releases the vitamin over an 8 to 10 hour period. It is very important that the maker of the tablet is legitimate in that there really is a sustained release of niacin. Some manufacturers have done studies to prove their claims. Ask about it before you buy.

EPA & DCA - No Fish Story

There are two important series of polyunsaturated fatty acids known to have vital biological functions. They are the Omega-3 series and the Omega-6 series.

EPA (eicosapentaenoic acid) is a precursor of the important prostaglandin 3 family (such as PGI-3). DHA (docosahexaenoic acid) is an important brain component. Together, they play an important role as a supplement to a total dietary program to reduce total fat consumption and to help reduce serum cholesterol to a manageable level.

Prostaglandins are remarkable biochemical regulators (similar to hormones).

In order to fully understand the function of fatty acids and their role in the production of prostaglandins, the following explanation is presented.

In a healthy human, linoleic acid (found in vegetable oils) is converted into gamma linolenic acid (GLA), then to dihomo gamma linolenic acid and finally to arachidonic acid. Arachidonic acid is the starting point for the production of one group of prostaglandins, PGI-2 and TXA-2 thromboxane.

Linolenic acid (notice the difference in spelling from linoleic acid) also from vegetable oils is converted in a series of steps into eicosapentaenoic acid (EPA) which, in turn, becomes PGI-3 and TXA-3.

Blood platelets, the blood structural component which can influence blood clotting, tend to clump together depending on the influence of various prostaglandins. By clumping together they begin to form a clot.

This is good when we cut ourselves and need the blood to clot.

This is not good if it happens inside a blood vessel.

Nature balances things if we give her the raw materials. PGI-2 tends to prevent clumping and TXA-2 conversely tends to promote clumping. This keeps clumping from going on in the wrong place at the wrong time but enables it to clot where it is needed.

However, for the system to remain in balance, PGI-3 and TXA-3 perform similarly and the four substances help to keep the body in maximum good health.

However, if there is a short supply of EPA then not as much PGI-3 can be manufactured and not as much TXA-3 can be manufactured. This upsets the balance and, as a result, the blood becomes more viscous (thicker) and clots tend to form more easily.

Other relationships follow when there is sufficient EPA available to the body.

Cholesterol levels are lowered.
Triglyceride levels are lowered.
HDL cholesterol levels are raised.
LDL cholesterol levels are lowered.
VLDL cholesterol levels are lowered.

How Do You Get This EPA?

Since a lot of this knowledge came about by studying the diet of Greenland Eskimos in the early 1970's, you might want to emulate their diet and eat 1/2 to 1 pound of mackerel or some other oily fish every day or two. This is not very likely when we consider the average American diet.

The alternative is to eat some fish like tuna or salmon, and to take capsules which contain fish oil.

When you take fish oil (EPA & DHA), the body does not have to go through the complicated procedure of converting dietary raw material into EPA.

Cod Liver Oil is a traditional fish oil that many Americans have come to know and to dislike for its fishy taste. However, Cod Liver Oil is not the oil of choice for EPA. The large amounts of Cod Liver Oil which would have to be taken to get a sufficient amount of EPA would simply provide too much vitamin A and D for safety.

Fish oil capsules can be swallowed easily and have no taste. Recommended dose is 2 capsules with meals.

Vitamin C

Vitamin C helps trigger the enzyme that breaks down cholesterol and triglycerides into free fatty acids. This reduces the risk of fatty deposits sticking to the walls of your arteries and cutting off the flow of blood.

It also helps to reduce excess serum cholesterol in doses of 500 milligrams three times a day or with a good timed release product.

Vitamin C reduced cholesterol deposits in laboratory animals. According to experiments done by Dr. Emil Ginter and his colleagues, rats fed vitamin C showed 30 to 40 percent lower cholesterol deposits than control groups without supplemental vitamin C. In other words, cholesterol build-up in the arteries simply plunged.

Vitamin E

Dr. Robert London, M.D., Sinai Hospital, Boston, found that vitamin E was able to increase the amount of HDL cholesterol in the blood.

Vitamin E also reduces the oxidation of fatty acids in the blood and thereby increases the oxygen available to the muscles and other tissues.

Alfalfa

It supplies saponins, compounds that reduce the absorption of cholesterol from the intestinal tract. Reasearch indicates that saponins may lower total cholesterol significantly without reducing the protective HDL component.

Garlic

"Effect of an Odor-Modified Garlic Preparation on Blood Lipids," Lau, B.H.S. et al. *Nutrition Research* 7:139-149, 1987.

Four ml. of garlic liquid extract daily significantly lowered total cholesterol, VLD cholesterol, and triglycerides and increased HDL.

"Effects of Garlic Oil on Platelet Aggregation, Serum Lipids and Blood Pressure in Humans," Barrie, S.A., Wright, J.V., and Pizzomo, J., E. J. *Orthomolecular Medicine.* 2 (1): 15-21, 1987.

This double blind, placebo-controlled crossover study administered either a placebo or 18 milligrams of garlic oil (extracted from 9 grams of fresh garlic) to 20 volunteers. Plate aggregation, mean blood pressure and total cholesterol decreased significantly and serum HDL levels increased significantly in the treated groups.

R.C. Jain, Assistant Professor of Pathology, Faculty of Medicine, University of Benghazi, observed a decrease in total cholesterol after three weeks of eating 5 grams of crushed garlic daily.

Arun Bordia, M.D., Department of Cardiology, Rajasthan, India, reported a 17 percent decrease in serum cholesterol after six months when the essential oil of garlic was taken in a dose of .25 milligram per kilogram of body weight.

Garlic & Onions

American Journal of Clinical Nutrition. 1981 Vol. 34, 2100-03.

In a study by Bordia, patients were given 15 milligrams daily of garlic oil for six months. This dose, equivalent to an ounce of raw garlic cloves, reduced cholesterol levels significantly. Both garlic and onion are protective against excessive blood clotting and excess cholesterol.

Lecithin & Phosphatidyl Choline

Bestways, November 1982, in an article featuring Dr. Robert Downs, D.C. "If you have a circulatory problem and want to help yourself, Lecithin is good, EPA is better and phosphatidyl choline (in my opinion) is the best. The last two used together are almost miraculous!"

Further on in the article, Dr. Downs explains that lecithin is excellent for circulatory impairment problems because the choline factor in lecithin has the positive ability to break down fat. This ability is useful in the treatment of arteriosclerosis, a heart disease characterized by fat deposits in the wall of the arteries caused by an accumulation of the wrong type of cholesterol.

There's enough research out now to state emphatically that two substances — phosphatidyl choline and EPA (from fish oil) are tremendously effective in reducing cholesterol and triglyceride levels.

Any type of fat that needs to be emulsified, such as gallstones or fat deposits in the liver or gall bladder will be helped by the use of phosphatidyl choline.

Lecithin will help too — there's no doubt about it - but you're dealing with a 3 to 1 ratio. That means you need three times the amount of lecithin to equal one phosphatidyl choline.

Don't expect a miracle cure in a week! It will take six months to a year of concentrated effort and a circulation improvement program. (These are strong words and I agree with Dr. Downs. In fact, I agree so much that I've changed my cholesterol control routine to conform to his appraisal.)

Lecithin alone is thought to have the capacity to alter the chemistry of cholesterol. From that fact alone, it is apparent that lecithin is a very important subject to understand when discussing serum cholesterol.

The important constituent of lecithin is choline, a member of the B-Complex family of vitamins which is essential to the metabolism of fats, especially in the liver.

There are two definitions of lecithin. The biochemical
definition is "phosphatidyl choline." The food definition is "mixed
phosphatides," which includes, at most, 25 percent phosphatidyl
choline.

Depending on who you speak to or what you know about your
general state of health, which is highly individual, either take lecithin
capsules (two with each meal) or 1 tablet of phosphatidyl choline with
two or three meals.

Gingko Biloba

Longevity, Vol. II No. 3, Jan. 1988.

According to a study at the University of Leeds in England,
gingko biloba extract generates good free radical scavengers which
destroy the harmful byproducts of oxidation resulting in an increase
in the supply of oxygen. Additional oxygen helps to burn fats in the
body.

Recommended dose for older people is one to three capsules
daily.

Pectin

Some fibers are helpful in cases of constipation (wheat bran
for example) but it will not help lower serum cholesterol. On the
other hand, pectin can help to lower cholesterol levels. In fact, there
is evidence that a combination of pectin and vitamin C can help
reduce cholesterol levels up to 20 percent. (*Life Extension Update*,
Vol. I No. 2)

Pectin can be found in apples, oranges, cherries, tomatoes,
carrots and other produce. It seems to help remove cholesterol from
the digestive tract. So can oatmeal, oat bran, and legumes such as
brown beans and chickpeas.

The best advice for the average person is to eat a mix of all
different kinds of fiber, says David Klurfeld, Ph.D., assistant professor
of the Wistar Institute.

If you do not, for some reason, take the professor's advice then look for a supplement which contains various fiber products from a number of sources.

My Personal Cholesterol Control Program

1) I've modified my diet according to the best nutritional advice I can find. That is, less red meat and more poultry (without the skin) and more fish. More steamed vegetables, less refined carbohydrates and more complex carbohydrates.

2) I'm on an exercise program which includes walking at least two miles a day.

3) I take a lot of vitamins and minerals plus the following specific nutrients to control cholesterol:

2 capsules of fish oil with meals
1 capsule of odorless garlic with meals
1 tablet of phosphatidyl choline with meals (I use the brand called Phos-Cal which is 95 percent)

(I used to take two capsules of lecithin with meals but after finishing the research for this chapter I switched to PhosCal.)

P.S. If I'm eating out and can't quite control the cholesterol content of the meal, I take one or two phytosterol tablets before eating.

Conclusion

Beyond introducing you to the various natural means of controlling a potentially dangerous situation, I can't recommend a dosage or a program to any individual. You may choose for yourself or take the matter up with your nutritionally-oriented doctor, along with the question of a complete dietary regime and exercise routine for your particular situation.

CONCENTRATED
FAT-BURNERS

by Dr. William H. Lee

Diet Panic and Stress Panic

Why is it that many people can eat everything they want and still look like models strolling down a runway?

How much does heredity have to do with your weight?

Blame it on a slow metabolism? "It's my thyroid gland that keeps me fat!"

The truth is, many factors get together in your body to determine whether you'll be fat or skinny. And, you can't control your weight unless you learn all the facts, understand the whole story — and then change all the factors under your control.

There are products on the market that can help you. You won't need a doctor's prescription to buy them. They're available in every health food store and drugstore. However, you do have to know your own body in order to choose the product that will benefit you the most.

Here's a quick rundown on fat-facts and theories to help you begin to understand your own body.

The reason we get fat goes back fifteen thousand years or more. Humans were just beginning to evolve into the "modern" men and women of today. Life was hard, and most waking hours were spent in finding enough food to sustain life. Man did not know how to store food during the warm months, and, even if he did, storage facilities were limited to the back of a cave. The idea of drying grains and seeds so they would last over the winter months had not yet occurred to ancient tribes, and the fact that cold months and warm months happened with regularity was not yet fully understood.

In that beginning culture the only guarantee of getting through the winter was to acquire a heavy layer of body fat. Women, because they had to bear the young to keep the race from dying out, were usually fatter than the men.

There are fat women and skinny women, however, and genetics play the biggest part in how many fat cells you acquire at birth. If your ancestors were among the fattest in the cave, they survived the toughest winters and passed their genes on to succeeding generations, ending up with you.

Why did the skinny women survive that tough winter? Maybe they attracted the best hunter in the cave, or were able to sit nearest the fire, or maybe they lived in a more temperate zone.

Whichever, everyone is born with a designated number of fat cells according to an individual genetic plan.

And not only are these fat cells permanent, but you can add to them. If you are excessively heavy, your body will manufacture new fat cells. Like the ones you were born with, the new fat cells will never disappear. And, fat cells are designed to store fat.

But, does that mean, "Once Fat — Always Fat"?

Fat cells can be shrunk. Flattened out. Be made almost invisible.

First off, don't blame your obesity on your metabolism, that's only a crutch to make yourself feel better. You may have a slow metabolism, but it isn't your metabolism that's making you fat. It's your fat that's giving you a slow metabolism. Part of the problem is that you went on a very restricted-calorie diet and it stimulated certain responses in your body. For that explanation we have once again to go back fifteen thousand years.

Enter Diet Panic

Many of the problems we face in this day and age can be traced back to the fact that the human body has changed very little since the cave days. We still eat food, need sunlight, bear young, and live in caves (we call them apartments or houses). Although physically our environment does not resemble the world of our remote ancestors, our bodies are essentially the same, and react in a similar manner to many of the same problems.

One of the problems is the safety of the race. The "old brain," the one that controls our basic needs and desires — like safety, sex, anger, all of the so-called "primitive" emotions, is alive and well in our bodies and is very concerned about our health as individuals and about the health of our human race.

Normally, we enjoy a regulating mechanism, the "new brain," a "younger" brain, which evolved at a later period. The actual location of this regulator is in the hypothalamus and, when operating as it should, helps keep our weight at our "set point," the level at which we feel most comfortable.

This mechanism balances caloric input against energy output. If we eat too much at one meal it helps us eat less at the next meal, or it initiates exercise (an increase in energy output) to make up for the extra calories. When working well, it helps keep our weight constant — whether at normal weight or beyond it.

Then we decide to go on a diet! We cut our food intake drastically — from 3,500 calories of food to 1,200 calories of food. And Diet Panic sets in.

"Famine!" "Begin emergency procedures!"

Diet Panic results from a lack of nutrients. You understand that you want to lose weight. But your body only knows that it was used to getting a load of vitamins, minerals, trace elements, protein, fat, and carbohydrates, and now that plentiful supply has been reduced by more than half.

Diet Panic takes over metabolism and fat storage. The regulating mechanism is instructed to start storing more fat and using less energy so a greater proportion of the smaller amount of food you are now eating is stored away in the fat cells and less fat is burned for energy.

We can get around Diet Panic by using nutritional magic and some of the substances available to help soothe its anguish. But first, there's another problem you should be aware of. It's called Stress Panic. It's another legacy from our cave days and is also responsible for the way we lose or gain weight.

As humans were evolving back in those early days, a complex set of physiological reactions were built into the body to handle the effects of stress. Stress then usually arose from physical danger, with the threat of death at every turn. Early humans reacted to this stress with explosive action.

Our bodies today still respond without conscious thought. The lungs and heart rush extra oxygen to the muscles, the pupils dilate for better vision, the muscles tense up for exertion, and the bloodstream is flooded with special hormones. The liver releases glucose for energy, and fat for extra fuel is dumped from the fat cells.

This famous "flight or fight" reaction is designed to save our lives in times of stress or danger. Without this unconscious reflex action, mankind might not have been able to overcome primitive disasters.

As modern people we also are stressed, but the stress we face in our lives is seldom physical. Rather it can be a pile of unpaid bills, an audit by the IRS, an irate boss, or bumper-to-bumper traffic. Fighting or running seldom helps these problems. We usually just smile and suppress our feelings.

But fear and anxiety will trigger the same stress reactions, as if we had come face-to-face with a saber-toothed tiger! Heart rate and breathing still increase. Hormones are still released. Sugar and fat are still dumped into the bloodstream. And the body is still prepared for action.

That's when Diet Stress goes to work. When no action takes place to use up all those potential "fight or flight" substances, Diet Stress gathers them all up and, you guessed it, stores them all away as fat!

And do you know what stresses the body most? Dieting!

So now you know about the two factors that keep most diets from working: Diet Panic, with its fear of famine, and Diet Stress, with its reluctance to lose any nourishment.

All the popular diets call for drastic reductions in the amount of food you eat. And they suggest a lot of exercise. So you eat less, sweat a lot and drop a pound or two. Then Diet Panic and Diet Stress wake up and your're back where you started when you step on the scale — maybe you're even a pound or two heavier!

If eating less and sweating are the only answers to the diet problem, why are there so many hungry fat people bathed in perspiration?

This is not a diet text in the true sense of the word. In this chapter there will be no endless lists of foods to avoid, or foods you must eat, or calorie tables, or recipes. There will be none of that at all. Instead, what you will find booklet is how to get around the natural forces in your body that work against your losing weight.

There are many good diets presented in many good books. Concentrated Fat-Burners will be compatible with any intelligent weight-loss program and any good exercise program (both are necessary for weight loss).

There are nutritional aids that can come between you and Diet Panic and persuade Diet Panic to relax its dictatorial policy.

There are nutrients that can replace the ones spent by the body on ineffectual responses to stress.

There are methods to increase so-called Brown Fat at the expense of White Fat (Brown Fat burns up White Fat for energy).

Concentrated Fat-Burners presents all the products and separate substances that are available to you. Since people are individuals, there is not one product or substance alone that is superior to all of the others. What will work in one case may not in another; so, you may have to try one approach and then another to find the ideal one for you.

It's always a good idea to go to your nutrition-oriented doctor before you begin any diet, whether you're going to use the natural substances in this chapter, or any other weight-loss method.

Your doctor can advise you about exercise and your present physical condition, when to exercise, and how strenuous the exercise routine should be.

He or she can also advise when to increase the amount and the duration of the program.

The doctor, knowing your medical history can also advise the use of amino acids or advise against the use, since there are certain very rare cases where one or more of these food substances should be avoided in the amount here suggested. (See section at end on Contraindications.)

On the whole, amino acids are completely safe for the vast majority of people, but it pays to be cautious if you suffer from certain genetic conditions.

Appetite is in Your Mind
Better Living Through Brain Chemistry

Appetite, like sex, it is said, begins in the mind.

Examine love at first sight: strangers look at each other and are attracted. The attraction stimulates brain chemicals (neurotransmitters) and a rapturous feeling floods the body. They kiss! According to British researchers, the kiss is a "tasting" procedure where each person samples the other's semio-chemicals secreted by special glands in the mouth area. If they like the "taste" they go on to explore other activities until satiated.

Appetite also begins in the brain! The brain monitors all physical activities and requires an adequate amount of fuel (food) to keep the body running as it should. When fuel is low, the brain sends out commands to eat in the form of neurotransmitters of brain chemicals. When there is a sufficient amount of high-grade fuel in the body, the brain produces another neurotransmitter which tells the body to stop eating! True hunger and normal eating are the results of chemicals manufactured by the brain, as is feeling full and the command to stop eating. So — it should be possible to lose weight and control your appetite by resorting to chemical principles!

And it is. You can manipulate the neurotransmitters in your brain, and outwit Diet Panic. You can reach your dream weight without ever resorting to agonizing diets — or dangerous drugs and prescriptions.

Nutrients are different from drugs. A nutrient is a food substance that, in most cases, supplies either building blocks the body needs to make cells and tissue, or energy the body needs to keep its mechanism functioning.

Drugs, on the other hand, work on a particular organ or cell.

All healthy people, obese or otherwise, must have the same nutrients, whereas a drug would be recommended only if there is a particular disease or condition to be treated.

However, under special circumstances, when nutrients are taken in food or as supplements, they can give rise to important changes in the chemicals manufactured by the body. And that principle can mean the difference between the success or failure of your weight-loss program!

In early days, before the concept that nutrition is an important factor in daily living, we assumed that what we ate had little effect on brain function, since the adult brain contained its own means to synthesize chemicals according to need. Now it appears that neurotransmitter synthesis in the brain is not as autonomous as once believed. The type of food offered to the body as fuel, and its protein content, can influence the manufacture of those brain chemicals.

Protein, carbohydrates, and fats are three life-sustaining nutrients. Living cells are manufactured from protein. The other two nutrients supply energy.

The proteins you get from meat, milk, eggs, rice, and other sources are first fragmented in the digestive tract into the amino acids. All protein is composed of chains of amino acids, from only a few to thousands, linked together in specific ways and in as many patterns as can be imagined.

All food protein is broken down into the individual amino acids, which are then reassembled into patterns needed by the body. There are basically twenty-two amino acids. Eight of the twenty-two are growth and maintenance chemicals, and are absolutely essential constituents of an adequate diet. These eight cannot be manufactured by the body, but must be obtained either from food or supplements. All the others, called nonessential amino acids, can be made by the body cells from fats or carbohydrates combined with nitrogen.

The brain uses certain amino acids as raw material in the manufacture of brain chemicals. When these amino acids are obtained from food, they are carried to the brain, passing through the blood-brain barrier, a protective device that prevents unwanted substances from invading the brain area.

Since most amino acids derived from food approach the brain area in more or less equal amounts and have to use the same "ferry-molecules" to cross the barrier, there is usually not much more of one amino acid than another.

We can now load the dice in favor of natural appetite suppression in two ways: First, by coaxing the brain to manufacture more and more of a special little chemical — one that prevents the Diet Panic that stops the body from burning fat. Then we can go on and convince the brain to make more of the chemical that says we have had enough to eat. So we feel great. We feel full. And the fat is melting off our bodies like butter.

One of the problems with a low-calorie approach to dieting is feeling deprived and hungry. You may be getting an adequate amount of nutrients (if you are also taking supplementary vitamins and minerals) but the empty feeling and Diet Panic work against you. Nutritional manipulation of brain chemicals can change the situation and strengthen your resolve to lose weight. And the amino acids involved in this particular nutritional approach are available in supplement form at your health food store or drugstore.

Phenylalanine

This is one of the essential amino acids that can help you control your appetite without becoming depressed. It is 100 percent natural. Phenylalanine is found in many foods, particularly in meats and milk.   When it reaches the brain it is turned into a neurotransmitter (a chemical that is able to transmit signals between the nerve cells and the brain).

It would be nice if you could get it from food and eat yourself thin, there would be no obesity and no need for this chapter. The problem, though, is the competition between all the amino acids to get into the brain area. Foods contain a number of amino acids. Meats and dairy products contain all the essential amino acids and all of them are digested at the same time and approach the brain at the same time.

Because there is a more or less even distribution of the amino acids, there is normally an even effect on the production of brain chemicals, but if you want to exert control over your own weight, you have to do more than just cut down on food and increase the amount of exercise you do. You have to induce your brain to work with you and not be at the mercy of Diet and Stress Panic. And that can be done with nutritional magic! You will not be taking chemicals or drugs that are harmful; you will be using natural substances found in food, only in their concentrated form, as tablets or capsules, such as Phenylalanine.

What Does Phenylalanine Do?

First, we have to put an "L" in front of the phenylalanine to distinguish it from D-Phenylalanine. The "L" form is important because with almost all the amino acids you will use, it is the "L" form that works best in the body. Read the label on the supplement bottle to make sure you are getting the right form.

When L-phenylalanine is able to cross the barrier into the brain in a larger than normal concentration, it is turned into noradrenaline (norepinephrine) and dopamine, two neurotransmitters. These brain chemicals tend to tilt the mental mood toward excitement, alertness, sexual awareness, and also help the body control appetite. L-phenylalanine invites the release of a hormone called cholecystokinin (CCK), one of the body chemicals that is normally released to tell the brain we have had enough to eat and are "full."

If this chemical is released early enough, you can eat less without having hunger pangs. If you eat less, but eat "smart," you will have an adequate supply of nutrients and will be able to burn body fat for energy instead of just storing food away.

L-phenylalanine needs vitamins to be effective, particularly vitamins C and B-6 (pyrodoxine). It is important to be taking a good multiple vitamin/mineral formula when you diet.

Additional benefits from L-phenylalanine include help in the production of natural epinephrine, a hormone manufactured by the adrenal glands, useful as a body stimulant, and thyroxine, a hormone needed to regulate the metabolic rate of the body. You need help in the production of the natural hormone that raises the metabolic rate of your body. Well, here it is. The metabolic rate governs the pace at which the body operates and the speed with which it burns fat. A sluggish rate burns fat more slowly.

L-phenylalanine also plays an important part in overcoming the desire to eat when you are feeling "blue."

There are many over-the-counter drugs available to help suppress your appetite. Some of these widely advertised products contain a substance that sounds like L-phenylalanine but isn't. It's called phenylpropanolamine (PPA). It works by causing the release of noradrenaline in the brain the same way that L-phenylalanine does. It doesn't trick the brain into making more of the noradrenaline, however, so it loses its ability in a very short span of time.

L-phenylalanine, on the other hand, will work each time you use it. You do not lose the effectiveness after a few weeks.

To speed up the process, take L-phenylalanine before lunch and supper as well. However, once your desired weight is reached, reduce the dosage to 100 to 500 mg at night or in the morning, to help you maintain your weight.

Amino acids are natural substances, but once you are satisfied with your condition, it's best to return the control over neurotransmitters to your body. You should be able to then remain at your best weight through appetite control and exercise, but if you should have to resort to the use of amino acids again, you can do so with the same safety as before.

You Should Avoid Using L-phenylalanine:

If you suffer from high blood pressure. A few sensitive individuals may experience a rise in pressure even at the low doses suggested.

If you suffer from the genetic disease phenylketonuria (PKU).

If your doctor has prescribed a monoamine oxidase (MAO) inhibitor.

Take 100 to 500 mg with about 250 mg vitamin C, and 25 to 50 mg vitamin B-6 or a multivitamin and mineral supplement that contains both, at bedtime.

Take 100 to 500 mg with vitamins in the morning before breakfast with a full glass of water.

If the exciting quality of amino acid should interfere with sleep, either reduce the dose or eliminate the nighttime dose.

Not all people with high blood pressure have to avoid using L-phenylalanine. Most people will not find that it affects their pressure. I only bring it up to make sure that you will monitor your pressure if you suspect some deviation. Your doctor can help you make a decision by teaching you to use a blood pressure device so you can test yourself at home.

L-Tryosine

L-tryosine is another essential amino acid with all the brain-changing qualities of L-phenylalanine, but without the blood-pressure-raising side effect some sensitive people experience. And while L-tyrosine will produce the same brain chemicals as L-phenylalanine (L-tyrosine — noradrenaline — dopamine), it may not influence the production of CCK in the intestine. It does, however, decrease appetite, help overcome the "blues," improve mental alertness and ambition, and lead to a more positive outlook on life.

L-tyrosine is also found naturally in meat, dairy products, and eggs. Although it is not an essential amino acid, since it can be manufactured (with difficulty) in the body, it is one of the more important food factors concerned with brain chemistry.

Although L-tyrosine usually has no effect on blood pressure, it is wise to monitor its use anyway.

Take 100 to 500 mg with about 250 mg vitamin C, and 25 to 50 mg vitamin B-6, or a vitamin and mineral supplement that contains both, at bedtime or before breakfast.

Begin with the smaller dose of L-tyrosine and slowly increase it until you begin to feel the effect on your appetite. You may want to raise or lower the dose at your pleasure.

L-Glutamine

Through nutritional magic and by the use of L-glutamine, a form of glutamic acid which the brain consumes for energy, we can feed the brain and quiet its craving for sweets.

Because L-glutamine can cross the brain barrier easily, and the brain can take it and quickly convert it into glutamic acid, if you take L-glutamine in supplemental form the brain will be able to satisfy its hunger more easily.

Glutamic acid serves primarily as a fuel for the brain's operation and as a buffer against excess ammonia.

The relationship of glutamic acid to glucose (blood sugar) goes beyond the brain-fuel interrelationship. Since the brain can store only a small amount of glucose, it is very dependent on the second-to-second supply of blood sugar which may explain dizziness and other nervous symptoms that accompany hypoglycemia (low blood sugar).

The gray matter in the brain converts glutamic acid to a special compound that helps regulate brain cell activity. Thus, a shortage of L-glutamine in the diet, and of glutamic acid in the brain, can result in brain damage due to excess ammonia or a brain that cannot get into "high gear."

The stress of dieting can lead some people who are not necessarily fond of alcohol to drink a lot more than usual in an effort to control the stess they feel.

Also, since alcohol is metabolized very quickly, it is converted to brain fuel, and during your diet your brain can feel hungry and ask for a drink. If you answer its request and continue to do so you can do more than just wreck your diet program.

Dr. Roger Williams, along with his colleagues at the Clayton Foundation for Research at the University of Texas, made the vital discovery that not only did L-glutamine protect against the poisonous effects of alcohol; it also controlled or stopped completely the craving for it.

L-glutamine is a versatile amino acid that can contribute to your diet program if, on your way to your best weight level, you suffer from any of the problems described.

Take L-glutamine (*not* glutamic acid) to help control an "irresistable" craving for sweets. Begin with a 200 mg capsule or tablet three times a day for one week. Then increase the dose to two capsules or tablets three times a day for one week.

If you feel more alert, more energetic, and have lost your craving for sweets or alcohol, you can then experiment with the amount of L-glutamine you take until you find the best level for you.

Dehydroepiandrosterone (DHEA)

A little-known hormone with an almost unpronounceable name, dehydroepiandrosterone (DHEA), may be the answer to a dieter's prayer. It can be a fountain of youth and miracle weight reducer.

Imagine being able to lose weight without altering your diet. This may be the result gathered from experiments begun by a research biochemist at Temple University's Fels Research Institute in Philadelphia.

Dr. Arthur G. Schwartz holds a doctorate in microbiology from Harvard University and post-doctoral fellowships at both Oxford University and the Albert Einstein College of Medicine in New York City. He recently discovered that a particular hormone (DHEA) is produced in the body in very large quantities up until the mid-20s, and then begins decreasing at a steady rate as the body ages.

It appears that this Concentrated Fat-Burner blocks an enzyme that the body uses to produce glucose. If the body can't process the sugar, it can't store it either.

Dr. Schwartz proposed that it increases the body's ability to transform food directly into energy. This enables the body to 'burn off' old excess fat — and prevent new fat from accumulating in the first place.

Schwartz's controlled experiments confirmed that DHEA will cause obese mice to lose weight even as they continue eating their regular menu and without the addition of any appetite-controlling substances. The mice eat normally. It's just that the calories are then converted to heat rather than fat, thereby allowing the animals to lose weight!

Other research suggests that DHEA may have stress-reducing properties as well as weight-reducing properties. Dr. Norman Applezweig, a biochemist, dreams that DHEA may reduce the diseases of aging and perhaps even prolong life. Applezweig says that he believes that DHEA slows down hormones that cause premature-aging factors in the body, thereby slowing down the aging process itself.

DHEA is hard to find in the marketplace, however. It is a natural hormone whose medical uses have already been reported and publicized. And since it cannot be patented, it would be foolish to spend the millions of dollars necessary for testing if the company testing could not recoup its investment and make a profit.

But, there is a member of the vegetable kingdom, the same Mexican yam that provided the steroids for the first birth control pill, that appears to be an abundant source of DHEA.

DHEA is not approved by the FDA, even as a nutritional supplement, but it has been incorporated into a few weight-reducing formulas available at some health food stores.

You'll have to be a detective and read labels carefully, but with perseverance and by asking questions you can find DHEA.

The Fat-Burners

Fats are the most concentrated energy source in the diet. When they are "burned" (combined with oxygen), they enable the body to function on all levels. There are many natural substances to "burn off" fat.

The more efficient the burning, the more energy is released, and the more fat is used up. Therefore, if obesity is being fostered by inefficiency in the fat-burning mechanism, and if that can be corrected easily with a dietary supplement, then a program of exercise, reduced caloric intake, and the use of that supplement should result in a new, slim person.

Coenzyme Q-10

Coenzyme Q-10, present in almost every cell in the body, has a structure similar to that of vitamin K, and helps to produce energy in the cells.

Since most cellular functions are dependent on the availability of energy, coenzyme Q-10 is essential for the health of all human tissues and organs. Although it can be manufactured in the body, deficiencies of the substance have been reported in a wide range of conditions, including obesity.

The tendency to become overweight may be associated in some cases with a certain metabolic makeup that results in decreased heat production. Many scientists now believe that most people do not gain weight because they eat too much. Instead, they gain weight because their bodies work against their efforts to diet — putting the pounds in storage rather than burning them.

During tests, serum coenzyme Q-10 levels were found to be low in 52 percent of the obese subjects tested. When they were given 100 mg of coenzyme Q-10, along with a calorie-restricted diet, there was a mean weight loss of thirty pounds in eight weeks.

Coenzyme Q-10 is generally well-tolerated, and no serious adverse effects have been reported. However, it is not recommended during pregnancy and lactation, or in the cases of known hypersensitivity. The FDA considers it to be only a food supplement, and it is not recognized for weight control.

Coenzyme Q-10 comes in 10 mg capsules or tablets. Try taking one capsule three times a day and vary the dose until you find the most appropriate dose for you. Usually two capsules three times a day is the top dosage for most people.

Gamma-Cryzanol (GO)

Many dieters are taking a page from the body-beautiful people. Weight lifters who want to keep their muscles up and their fat down have found a white powder called gamma-cryzanol, extracted from rice bran oil. If you want to develop a slim, strong, athletic-looking figure, this may be your best — and easiest — bet.

It increases lean body mass, decreases fatty tissue, helps fight the energy loss brought on by dieting, and may help relieve the stress symptoms that accompany menopause.

Although it was discovered more than thirty years ago by a Japanese researcher, it only recently came to the attention of body builders trying to get more out of their workouts. They found that gamma-cryzanol (called GO) was an ergogenic aid, a work-enhancing, energy-producing substance that fights the energy drain of dieting.

GO probably works on the hypothalamus in the brain which, through its control of the pituitary gland, governs a number of your body's automatic functions, including temperature control, water balance, and hormonal regulation. Those hormones include the sex hormones — testosterone in the male and estrogen in the female.

It appears that GO may increase testosterone production. This may be the reason for an increase in lean body mass that researchers have observed when laboratory animals were fed a diet supplemented with this nutrient.

Researchers have also observed that fatty tissue appears to decrease when GO is used as a supplement in conjunction with controlled caloric intake and an exercise program. It might also benefit women in ways besides dieting. There have been controlled experiments in which GO administered to women has brought about a blessed reduction of the painful symptoms of menopause — without the slightest need for hormones or drugs.

There are some formulas on the market that combine GO with some of the other antioxidant and protective nutrients.

Take 5 mg daily. If you do heavy exercise, you can take up to 15 mg daily. The FDA has not authorized GO as anything but a nutritional supplement.

Phosphosugar

This compound of sugar and phosphorus is a basic source of energy to the body when combined. Every body cell must have energy to live and carry on its work. Without phosphosugar, the energy release would not be possible.

Most dieters go on a low-carbohydrate diet which interferes with the energy level and reduces the ability to concentrate, exercise, and do work of any sort. The brain, feeling overly tired, sends out the command to eat more carbohydrates, thereby interfering with the continuation of the diet.

Under normal conditions, persons eating a well-balanced diet will derive phosphosugar from their food sources. However, dieters, by reducing carbohydrate intake, will deplete themselves of their carbohydrate and fat reserves.

This is done on purpose, as a way to lose pounds. When carried to an extreme, carbohydrate reduction forces the body to break down amino acids for energy. If the intake of protein is also inadequate, the body may break down its own protein, including the protein that goes to make up the muscles.

If the intake of phosphorus is inadequate, the body may even rob the bones of their phosphorus content. Therefore, your diet must consist of at least one meal a day containing adequate amounts of protein, plus fresh vegetables to prevent breakdown of protein.

Phosphosugar is not fattening because the sugars in it are glucose and fructose (monosaccharides). Glucose is the primary source of energy for humans. The excess over what the body uses for energy is not turned into fat but glucose is not metabolized unless it is first bound to phosphorus.

Fructose is a fruit sugar that produces glycogen and maintains normal content of glucose in the blood. In the liver, it may be converted into glycogen, which in turn may be converted into glucose.

Phosphosugar contains the ingredients needed by the body to make ATP, which fuels your cells. This product may be hard to find since all health food stores do not stock it. When you do locate it, follow manufacturer's directions. Usually you would use it twice a day, say before breakfast and before lunch. It comes in small packets and should be mixed with a citrus juice. It has a slightly bitter tast, even though it sounds as if it ought to be sweet. The FDA has not approved this product as a diet aid.

Carnitine

L-carnitine is the fat-burner that works at your body's deepest level — without any help from your will power!

Recent research indicates that L-carnitine, one of the amino acids, plays an important role in converting stored body fat into energy.

In its action with the cell's engine (the mitochondrion), which burns fat for energy, carnitine accelerates the rate at which the body burns fat. The more fat that is burned — the less you have to carry around with you. So, the more carnitine, the more fat your body can burn, and the more energy you get from your body.

It is also important in controlling hypoglycemia, energizing the heart, reducing the effects of angina attacks, and is beneficial to patients suffering from diabetes, liver disease, or kidney disease.

The food sources of L-carnitine are meat and dairy products but the amounts found in these foods are not enough for weight loss.

Therefore, supplements of L-carnitine should be taken in a 250 mg tablet twice daily; however, if there is any evidence of allergy (people can be allergic to anything, even water) the use of L-carnitine alone should be discontinued and the use of a combination with other substances should be considered. The FDA does not consider L-carnitine to be anything but a food supplement.

Trade in Fat for Muscle

For years all you've been told is "the only way to lose weight is to eat less," but dieting is an unscientific way to lose weight! However, a cure for obesity may be just around the corner.

About ten years ago, give or take, researchers discovered the presence of a special hormone in the human body. They named it "Human Growth Hormone" (HGH).

What was curious about this substance is that when it was given to animals, they were able to eat huge amounts of food without growing fat. In fact, they ended up in better physical condition than before they began the test.

Someone began to speculate about friends of theirs — lean, hungry, thin people who eat huge amounts of food but seldom vary their weight more than a couple of pounds either way.

When they investigated further, they discovered that the HGH levels in lean people were higher than the HGH levels in obese people.

According to Pearson and Shaw, in their book *Life Extension*, "Growth hormone causes one to put on muscle and burn fat. Everyone knows that most teenagers eat like horses without becoming obese, even if they are sedentary. A middle-aged person eating the same food and getting the same exercise will usually become fat. The higher growth hormone levels in teenagers have a great deal to do with the difference."

HGH is stored in the pituitary gland in all healthy people of all ages. One of its purposes is to make sure that during the growing years, fat can be converted into fuel and muscle tissue to serve the needs of the growing body.

As we age, however, the release of HGH slows down and by the age of thirty (not old by any means), the flow has virtually ceased, perhaps because older people need the extra amount of fat to stay warm, and as extra fuel in case there is a shortage of food (a body system set up eons ago to help people survive in caves, not in today's world).

But when you diet (remember that the body thinks in terms of famine), the body does not respond by released HGH. It does just the opposite, it hoards the fat. The more you starve yourself, the more your body fights you!

Therefore, it is necessary to bypass the diet and go directly to HGH release.

In June of 1982, Pearson and Shaw said, "The amino acids L-arginine and L-ornithine, taken on an empty stomach at bedtime, cause growth hormone release by increasing the basal metabolic rate and burning off fat during sleep. These can easily make a normal 65-year-old's growth hormone levels resemble those of a teenager."

It's best to take it at night, since HGH release occurs within the first ninety minutes of sleep. During the night, while you are soundly sleeping, the HGH can safely burn off ounces of fat.

For the best results, these amino acids should be used in combination with a balanced, medium-calorie diet, daily exercise, and proper sleep.

Most health food stores and drugstores stock various combinations and individual amino acids. They usually combine twice the amount of L-arginine as L-ornithine.

Take 500 mg L-arginine and 250 mg L-ornithine. The instructions are usually on the bottle. Take one or two at night before bedtime.

Another formula combines the following: L-arginine 1200 mg, L-ornithine, 900 mg, L-lysine 1200 mg. Take one or two at bedtime.

While still another formula acts to combine the L-arginine and L-ornithine with vitamin B-3, vitamin B-6, and the amino acid L-tryptophan. Again, the directions are to take them at night.

The FDA does not recognize any of these formulas as diet aids.

Feel Full With Fiber

Fiber provides bulk without calories and can perform other beneficial acts in the body.

The two best fibers are natural materials. One, called glucomannan, is derived from a plant root and the other is a micro-algae called spirulina.

Glucomannan has been used in Japan for centuries, and spirulina has been a food source in Africa for at least that long. Both of them are very low in calories. Both are high in fiber. Both absorb water and create a feeling of fullness in the stomach. Both have a history of safety extending back thousands of years.

Both are available at health food stores or at drugstores at only a fraction of the cost of prescription diet pills.

Spirulina

An ancient nutrient, which may have been the first active microorganism on earth, may be one of the best weapons against obesity. Only very recently has the weight-regulating ability of this food, a type of plankton, been understood and applied to a diet program.

Spirulina is a rare mine of vitamins and minerals. It is 60-70 percent digestible protein. It is a natural source of vitamin B-12 from the vegetable kingdom which is usually found only in food of animal origin. It is a recognized source of Beta-carotene, which the body converts into usable vitamin A. It contains the B-complex vitamins, plus substantial amounts of iron and other minerals. It is also a source of mucopolysaccharides, essential unsaturated fatty acids, nucleic acids, chlorophyll, plus some vitamin E.

It is available in most health food stores and in some drugstores. You can buy it in tablet form, as a powder, as a diet formula, energy food, pasta, and as flakes to sprinkle on other foods. It is also included in stress-reducing supplements offered for sale in some health food stores.

You can adjust the dosage to suit your own individual needs. Try taking three of the 500 mg tablets (or the equivalent in any other form) with a full glass of water one-half hour before meals.

If this is the right dosage for you, and it succeeds in reducing your hunger or keeping it away, try reducing the amount to two tablets or even one tablet before meals. The FDA has permitted it to be imported into this country as a food supplement, but has not classified it for any other purpose.

Glucomannan

Supplementing your diet with glucomannan not only makes good scientific sense, it also has a history of safety that goes back over two thousand years.

Glucomannan is derived from the edible root of the konjac plant (amorphophallus konjac), which is in the same family as the yam. The Japanese have long cultivated and reaped the benefits of this plant.

The glucomannan gently swells in the stomach, bringing a feeling of fullness. When the stomach feels full, it sends a signal to the hypothalamus (the appetite-control center). The hypothalamus then, in turn, sends a return signal to reduce hunger and appetite. Because of the feeling of fullness and the presence of supplemental nutrients provided by the vitamin tablets you take, Diet Panic and Diet Stress do not set in.

People who follow this simple diet technique eat less food during meals and feel satisfied much more quickly. But since it speeds the transit of the food through the stomach, it cuts down on the amount of nutrients the body can absorb in that shorter space of time. All this is a help to you as far as losing weight, but you have to be careful not to cut down on nutrition.

Therefore, it is suggested that you have one meal a day without the use of the glucomannan. Take your vitamins with this meal as well, to insure absorption of the supplemental nutrients.

Some people can feel a bit bloated when they begin to use glucomannan. If that happens, just cut the dose in half for two or three days to let your system adjust to it.

In most health food stores it is available in powder, capsule, cake, tablet, cookie and candy forms. Glucomannan expands fifty to sixty times in size when it reaches the stomach. The idea is to take about 1,000 mg. Usually it comes in 500 mg capsules or tablets, so take two with eight ounces of water one-half hour before a meal.

Glucomannan is offered for sale as a dietary supplement and has not been approved by the FDA for any other purpose.

Food Fiber

Hunger and the need to eat are normal body mechanisms controlled by our most primitive brain, which can supersede the more modern brain under crisis conditions.

The desire to eat is as strong as urge as your sex drive. Because you need to eat to stay alive, your empty stomach will nag at you with hunger pangs, rumbling, growling, and gas attacks.

In order to stop this reminder that your stomach demands filling, you have to put something in it or you will be bullied into eating. Filling your stomach is the job of substances like glucomannan, spirulina, and our western counterpart, fiber!

Bran fiber, for one, is the tough outer coating of the cereal grain. While it and other cereal grain fibers do not possess glucomannan's amazing power to swell in the stomach, fiber does make you feel full and less hungry when taken before a meal in supplement form or as part of a meal.

Fiber has the ability to modify hunger and cleanse the digestive tract of toxins.

Fiber is defined as the undigestible cell walls of plants. It has been called roughage, bulk, plant residue, plantix, and unavailable carbohydrates. The medical profession defines fiber as dietary components that increase fecal bulk, or those parts of plant materials which are resistant to digestion by secretions of the human gastrointestinal tract.

Fiber includes cellulose, hemicellulose, lignins, pectins, gums, mucilages, and storage polysaccharides. The majority of plant fibers (such as cellulose, hemicellulose, and lignin) are insoluble and play their part in the health of the body due to their insolubility.

Pectins, on the other hand, can be digested or fermented in the colon.

Consider the effect of eating an apple compared to drinking some apple juice. It's the pectin in the whole apple that helps you feel satisfied. The juice, which is devoid of pectin, can never give you the feeling of fullness that the whole apple can.

Most nutritionists recommend at least 30 to 45 gm of assorted fiber a day. That's a difficult amount to ingest, since, for example, 1 slice of whole wheat bread only has 2 grams, as does 1 small banana and a small potato.

Fiber supplements are available in health food stores in a number of forms. There are fiber tablets, fiber wafers, fiber crackers, fiber candy bars, fiber soups, and so on. A good fiber supplement will combine fibers from an assortment of foods. Look for pectin and various fruit fibers on the label.

If you want to use the fiber tablets, wafers, or crackers, chew them very well and make sure that you drink at least eight ounces of water with them.

Two or more tablets, wafers, or crackers one-half hour before meals with water is the usual dose.

There may be a bit of stomach growling or distension if you are not used to having fiber in your system. If this happens, reduce the amount you are taking for two or three days and then begin again.

More Efficient Prostaglandins
Gamma-linolenic Acid (GLA)

Some say a new era of diet control is here, thanks to the natural magic of a substance called gamma-linolenic acid (GLA).

It seems that GLA is a substance that calms Diet Panic. It restores you to your benevolent self and starts your body burning fat.

Scientists have long suspected that everybody has some kind of fat-burning mechanism, and now they have discovered that it comes in two parts. The first is the special kind of tissue called Brown Fat, less than 1% of the total weight of the average human and brown in color. This makes it different from the fat the body burns, which is White Fat. The reason Brown Fat is brown is that it is loaded with large numbers of fat-burning motors, known as mitochondria. It is in these motors that White Fat is burned and excess calories are consumed, instead of being stored away in fat cells. Under normal circumstances, when you eat, the brain tells your Brown Fat to burn off the extra calories.

Researchers have discovered that thin people have active and well-functioning Brown Fat, but overweight people have Brown Fat with a low level of fat-burning activity.

This means that the Brown Fat in overweight people is not cooperating, not burning up the extra calories the way it should. And, since the calories aren't burned, the body has no choice but to store them away in the fat cells.

Cool temperatures in the range of 65 or 66 degrees Fahrenheit are thought to activate Brown Fat. You need to be cold, but not cold enough to shiver. If you shiver, then the activity in the Brown Fat will decrease.

Exercises that do not increase body temperature will cause an increase in Brown Fat. Try swimming in luke-warm water.

The other part of the fat-burning mechanism is a system called the "sodium pump." This system regulates the amount of sodium and potassium (essential minerals) that are in the body cells.

Thin people tend to have sodium pumps that work properly and efficiently, burning large numbers of calories. Overweight people have defective pumps that don't do their jobs very well and burn a lot fewer calories. It is possible that many people, if not most, do not gain weight simply because they eat too much. Their bodies work against them, putting the pounds in storage instead of burning them.

The important thing is not how many calories you take in but how your body processes them.

So, if you're counting on calorie reduction to do the trick, and your body has lost its ability to burn up the few calories you do eat, it will still store fat no matter how restricted the diet!

GLA is one of the natural aids you'll need to burn up fat but it is hard to find in the foods you normally eat.

Oil of Evening Primrose

An excellent source of GLA, scientists have found, is oil of evening primrose. It is native to the United States, and the American Indians knew about it and its medicinal properties. They used it to treat skin diseases and inflammation, to drain bloating out of the body, to heal wounds, and to help those with asthma. The root was used as a sedative and a cough suppressant, it also was used as a pain killer and an astringent.

The Pilgrims soon discovered its medicinal use and quickly transported seeds to England where it was known as a panacea. It was so venerated that it became known as the "King's Cure-All."

The most recent results of the use of evening primrose oil capsules come from the Department of Nutrition at the Tulane University School of Public Health in New Orleans, Louisiana.

Evening primrose oil was given for six weeks to twenty-three overweight individuals, one or both of whose parents was also obese. When the results were in, compared to a control group taking placebo capsules, those taking evening primrose oil capsules had demonstrated a significant weight loss even though calorie intake actually rose.

Moreover, activity of the sodium pump increased in the group taking evening primrose oil, but not in the group taking the placebo capsule.

Evening primrose oil is usually available in 500 mg capsules at health food stores.

But, don't rush out and buy them! There's a better way to get GLA. Evening primrose oil contains about 9 percent GLA, but now there's a product on the market that contains about 18 percent GLA. Many companies package it. Ask for GLA and read the label carefully. This, too, is available in your health food store.

Follow the directions on the bottle. Take six capsules daily (two with each meal). Check the label to make sure that each capsule contains at least 40 mg of GLA (240 mg daily).

Include a vitamin and mineral supplement that will supply at least: 1000 mg vitamin C; 25 mg zinc; 100 mg B-6; 50 mg B-2; 50 mg B-3 (niacinamide).

Cholesterol Control

Although cholesterol, in excess, is a problem to all people, it is a greater problem to the obese.

Cholesterol is a white waxy fat required for membrane structures in all animals and humans, and is the starting material for the synthesis of many important hormones in the body, including the sex hormones, cortisone, and others.

Cholesterol is so essential that the human body could not survive without it — which is probably the reason why every cell in the body can manufacture it. Everyone is capable of producing all of the cholesterol needed by the body.

Since coronary artery disease and heart attacks are directly related to blood-cholesterol levels, the more cholesterol you eat in your diet, the greater your chance of having a heart attack and dying.

Your chances of suffering from this disease are lessened by eating a diet that contains no cholesterol. But, unless you are a strict vegetarian who eats no meat, dairy products, or eggs, it is virtually impossible to completely eliminate cholesterol from the diet because it is found in all dietary products that begin with animals.

Cholesterol threatens life mainly by contributing to atherosclerosis which is the underlying disorder in most coronary heart disease and, in addition, plays a major role in cardiovascular disease (stroke).

During a ten year period ending in 1984, the National Heart, Lung and Blood Institute (NHLBI) studied what relationship, if any, existed between cholesterol and heart disease. The results of this investigation, involving over 3,800 male subjects, are quite revealing. A principal finding of this study showed that the risk of heart attack deaths dropped 2 percent for every 1 percent reduction in serum cholesterol.

It is clear that cholesterol absorption is proportional to cholesterol ingestion.

However, nature has provided us with sensible and easy ways to reduce the absorption of the cholesterol component in these good-tasting foods. They're called phytosterols which are natural cousins to cholesterol found in the plant kingdom, mostly in grains, nuts, seeds, and fruit. Among the various types of phytosterols that exist, three have been found to be of the greatest nutritional importance. They are called: beta-sitosterol, stigmasterol, and campesterol.

Their natural distribution is in the common oils, corn, wheat, peanut and sunflower. You can avoid the extra calories, however, by getting a concentrate of natural sterols in tablet form.

The majority of the scientific evidence gathered from animal and human studies suggests that phytosterols consistently delay and reduce the absorption of dietary cholesterol into the circulation.

In other words, when phytosterols and cholesterols are combined during a meal, a certain percentage of the cholesterol will be blocked from the blood stream and forced to leave the body along with the waste material.

These tablets can be found in health food stores and drugstores. A daily intake of at least 300 mg (based on the beta-sitosterol content of the tablets) taken with meals (because it must be present along with the cholesterol) can have a significant effect on serum cholesterol.

But, you can't rely on the tablets alone! You have to do a little cutting back on cholesterol-laden foods along with it. That means more vegetables, fruits, less meat and dairy products.

Other cholesterol fighters that should be included in your diet include: fiber, fish and fish oils, garlic and onions, avocado oil, and, of course, a good exercise program.

The FDA has not commented on the ability of phytosterols to lower serum cholesterol.

Glucose Tolerance Factor, Insulin, and Body Fat

The role of glucose tolerance factor (GTF) in body fat appears to indicate that anyone having a weight problem should concentrate on reducing with the aid of high quality foods rich in GTF, and should use GTF in supplement form.

GTF is a vital compound that helps control blood sugar. This new supplement can be good news for millions of people who have a craving for sweets.

One of the major components of GTF is chromium, the shiny stuff on car bumpers. But, in the human body, chromium has the critical role of working with insulin to allow body cells their regular flow of glucose. Chromium is crucial, irreplaceable, and often overlooked as an essential nutrient.

Of all the trace minerals we need for good health (zinc, calcium, potassium, selenium and so on), only chromium gradually disappears as we mature.

GTF can be absorbed directly from food. Foods such as brewer's yeast (the richest source), mushrooms, wheat germ, oysters, certain cheeses, whole wheat bread, liver, corn oil, beets, fresh fruit, and chicken breasts contain small amounts, but only about 1 percent of dietary chromium is absorbed.

A deficiency can arise either because GTF is not in the food you eat, or you can't put the pieces together efficiently. The aging process also causes a significant decrease in GTF in many people.

GTF chromium is removed when food is refined. It is unfortunate that the further we remove food from the way nature meant it to be, the more problems we create for ourselves.

During experiments to discover the structure of GTF, it was learned that GTF significantly decreased cholesterol and triglycerides in diabetic and chromium-deficient animals.

The reversal of cholesterol deposits is accomplished by lowering the blood cholesterol and increasing high density lipoprotein (HDL) — the cholesterol carrier that scavenges cholesterol and carries it back to the liver for disposal.

There are two cholesterol ferries in the body. One, called low density lipoprotein (LDL), delivers cholesterol around the body and the other, HDL, removes it from the body. The higher the ratio of HDL to LDL, the less chance of heart trouble.

Said one writer: The more garbage trucks (HDL) you have than delivery trucks (LDL), the better condition your arteries will be in and the fewer problems you'll have with plaque.

Tests cited in the *American Journal of Clinical Nutrition*, November 1980, link chromium deficiency with atherosclerosis, coronary heart disease, obesity, and hypoglycemia.

You can get tablets of GTF at your health food store or drugstore. Normal maintenance levels run about 500 mcg a day.

Help From the Land and From the Sea

Kelp

Kelp is a remarkable food containing more mineral matter and vitamins than many well-advertised proprietary health foods, with the added advantage of being grown in the sea without the addition of artificial fertilizers.

Kelp acts on obesity mainly through the thyroid gland, which it tends to normalize. Thyroid gland malfunction, even on a small scale, can contribute to obesity on one hand or to extreme thinness on the other hand. Hence, a normal thyroid helps to maintain normal weight.

It has been determined that there is a definite connection between our energy and our intake of iodine. In kelp we have a perfectly natural source of all the iodine we need.

Not only does kelp help heal a problem thyroid, but it also has a healing and normalizing effect on the nervous system, arteries, colon, liver, gall bladder, and fat cells.

Kelp is available in tablets and granules at health food stores and in drugstores. (Comment: if you suspect that your weight problem is due to an underactive thyroid gland you must check first with your doctor. He may prescribe tablets containing thyroid or a synthetic compound that acts to stimulate thyroid function.) Follow manufacturer's directions for dosage.

Chlorella

There is a small, one-celled algae called chlorella that is a powerhouse of proteins, vitamins, and minerals. It contains more chlorophyll than any other edible plant, and contains 60 percent good-quality protein.

Frequently, dieters are in need of a detoxification process, some way to get rid of accumulated waste material. Chlorophyll is well known for its detoxification abilities.

A person doesn't have to wait long after taking chlorella to discover its detoxification properties. Within a few days the bowels begin to function much better than before.

Chlorella is rich in nutrients and protein. It is useful as part of a weight-loss program. When used as such it should be taken with at least eight ounces of water. Meals should consist, for the most part, of vegetables, cereals, salads, and fruits.

Chlorella is stocked in health food stores and drugstores. Use it according to manufacturer's instructions for best results.

Wheat Grass

This grass is high in fiber and protein. It contains chlorophyll and other nutrients characteristic of deep green, leafy vegetables. We should supplement our diets with green roughage foods like concentrated, dehydrated wheat grass, or barley.

Besides being a concentrated source of the nutrients associated with green leafy vegetables, wheat grass is high in fiber. When taken before meals with a large glass of water, it expands at least fifteen times its original volume in the stomach to help you feel full. This enables you to control your appetite and consume less food at each meal.

Wheat grass tablets do not contain sugar. Use four to ten tablets with each meal with a full glass of water. You can start by taking two tablets and gradually build up to a maximum of ten. Or, follow manufacturer's instructions.

Barley

Young barley leaves contain a juice that is a pleasant source of vitamins, minerals, and enzymes. According to an analysis made by the Resource Association Office of Science and Technology, and Japan Food Analysis Center, the juice contains thirty times as much vitamin B-1 as does milk, over three times as much vitamin C and six times as much carotene as does spinach. It has eleven times as much calcium as cow's milk, nearly five times the iron found in spinach, seven times the vitamin C in oranges, plus 80 mcg of vitamin B-12.

Its enzymes help digestion and loosening of hard fat. Its daily use helps solve a number of problems associated with obesity.

Barley can be found in health food stores in juice form, and in tablets or granules. Follow manufacturer's instructions for use.

Combined Nutrient Formulas and Other Aids
Nutrient Formulas

Many combinations of nutrients are available on the market, and most of them have some good points to offer to the dieter.

One formula combines papaya, garlic, and kelp. Natural foods can alter the body chemistry. Papaya contains a substance called papain. Papain, capable of splitting protein, is considered to be an aid to digestion and will affect the caloric measure of ingested food.

Garlic has been said to have an amazing number of benefits. One such is the ability to clear the bloodstream of collected fats. This fat-clearing process contributes to weight loss, in that fats will be carried away in your body's waste products and not stored in the cells.

Kelp is a natural source of iodine needed by the thyroid gland to govern the basic metabolic rate (the speed at which food is burned for energy). This formula of natural substances, when combined with a limited diet and an increase in exercise, can be of help to many people who want to lose a few pounds, but not necessarily for those who are more than 15 percent over their best weight.

Another combination of natural substances designed to keep your energy level up while the pounds go down utilizes bee pollen, octacosonal, spirulina, and ginseng. These four substances can give you energy without resorting to the use of artificial stimulants.

Bee pollen is one of the most effective energy foods known. It is a complete food, containing sixteen vitamins, sixteen minerals, eighteen enzymes, eighteen amino acids, and twenty-eight trace elements. All of the nutrients are balanced. It is a rich source of protein and energy.

Octacosanol is an important energy-releasing food substance derived primarily from wheat. Octacosanol has been shown to improve strength, endurance, glycogen storage, and the ability to utilize oxygen more efficiently.

Spirulina is a tiny freshwater plant (vegetable plankton) that may be nature's most perfect source of complete protein.

Ginseng is the famous herb that has been used for thousands of years to enhance both physical and mental energy levels and to increase endurance.

Still another formula combines the following: potassium chloride, L-tyrosine, glucomannan, grapefruit and octacosanol.

The enzymatic action of grapefruit on the body appears to start a fat-burning process that is boosted by the amino acid L-tyrosine (found in meat and cheese).

Glucomannan further suppresses appetite by virtue of its ability to expand in the stomach (provided a sufficient amount of water is taken with this formula), producing a feeling of fullness.

Potassium chloride is added to control excess fluids in the body and to also support the working of the adrenals.

Octacosanol, the ergogenic factor derived from wheat germ, is present to help put back the energy that dieters usually lose when the amount of food intake is restricted.

Some weight loss products utilize a substance called guar gum. Guar gum is a natural dietary fiber that can absorb up to sixty times its weight in water. Because it is not digestible, guar gum increases the bulk of matter in the stomach (provided enough water is taken with it). Studies show that guar gum can help reduce elevated serum cholesterol, another plus to obese individuals.

Guar gum speeds matter through the intestines and normalizes bowel functions. It is available separately in tablet or packet form or as part of a reducing formula with other substances. It can be found in health food stores and drugstores. Use as directed by the manufacturer.

Another formula consists of apple cider, vinegar, kelp, lecithin, vitamin B-6 and grapefruit extract.

The apple cider, vinegar, and lecithin work with the grapefruit extract to break down fat and cholesterol in the body. The combination of these four ingredients act as a gentle diuretic to help rid the body of excess water.

The next formula adds some amino acids: grapefruit, glucomannan, kelp, lecithin, apple cider vinegar, vitamin B-6,

L-tyrosine, and L-phenylalanine. They are in such a pure form that within thirty minutes they not only reduce hunger pangs, but also produce a hormone that "convinces" your brain that you've already eaten enough.

The next formula has double fiber: grapefruit concentrate, glucomannan, guar gum, vitamin C, L-phenylalanine, and L-tyrosine.

Try health food stores and drugstores for these formulas. Read labels and read directions carefully when you buy any reducing formula. Remember! If the label shows any type of fiber, you must have a sufficient amount of water to activate it. Drink at least eight ounces of water, and perhaps a bit more each time you take a dose. Follow manufacturer's instructions.

The Garcinia Cambogia Fruit

In Southeast Asia, researchers have come up with an interesting substance that is extracted from the rind of an edible fruit known as Garcinia cambogia (called the Brindall berry in the United States).

The berry contains natural fruit and fibers and the rind is a source of a substance called hydroxycitric acid that appears to be an effective adjunct to any weight loss program. The berry has been eaten for years in Asia without any harmful effect, and there have been toxicity studies done as well, which prove its harmless character.

Hydroxycitric acid is effective in reducing appetite and weight gain without having to resort to either stimulants or laxatives.

Also, when Brindall berry is used for dieting there is no "rebound" effect when it is discontinued. You never want to go on an eating binge.

And, it has been observed that hydroxycitric acid, because it inhibits fatty acid production, also reduces serum cholesterol and triglyceride levels up to 30 percent.

This is one product you may have to look for. Not all health food stores know about it and not all of them have it in stock. If you ask around, you will be able to find it.

Take one or two tablets before meals with a glass of water. Give the Brindall berry formula a chance to dissolve in the stomach

before you sit down to eat. The FDA has registered this product as
a dietary supplement and not as an aid to reducing.

Bee Pollen

For many centuries pollen has been esteemed as a valuable
nutrient in many corners of the world.

Devotees have voiced grandiose claims for bee pollen, calling
it a youth promoter and a nutrient-dense energizer for use during
dieting ("nutrient-dense" refers to the best ratio of nutrition to calories.
Exactly the opposite of "junk foods.") It is a perfectly-balanced food
containing all twenty-two amino acids, twenty-seven mineral salts, a
full range of known and unknown vitamins, and a collection of the
most needed enzymes. It has regenerative properties for the organism.
Its use in experiments with aging people seems to help restore morale,
a sense of spiritual well-being, and actual physical health. It firms
aging and lifeless skin. Among all age groups, many of the ailments
that responded favorably to bee pollen were chronic colitis, high blood
pressure and allergies.

Bee pollen pellets are found in health food stores and
drugstores, but pollen is expensive and small amounts are included in
many balanced diet formulas. If you want to buy pollen pellets and
use them with meals as an extra nutritional source, it depends a lot on
your pocketbook. Follow package instructions.

Octacosanol

By definition, octacosanol is an isolated, biologically active
factor of wheat germ oil. It is a natural ergogenic (energy-releasing)
substance that improves endurance, speeds up reaction time, provides
glycogen to muscles and strengthens them.

Octacosanol may increase fertility and prevent spontaneous
abortion, lower cholesterol and aid in the treatment of neurological
disorders.

It also appears to be extremely helpful in weight reduction,
through its ability to relax the nerves of your stomach to keep them
from tensing up and driving you crazy with hunger pains.

Octacosanol also increases the metabolic rate and reduces muscle tension.

Octacosanol is removed during the making of white flour but, even if processing didn't take it out of our food, we couldn't get the amount that is concentrated into supplement form. It would take over 4.5 million pounds of wheat to get just one pound of octacosanol.

Octacosanol may act as an aphrodisiac. It steps up production of semen in men and provides the extra energy needed for renewed passion. It is possible that octacosanol stimulates the pituitary gland, which controls almost everything that happens in the body.

Agility, total reaction time, and mental acuity can be helped by this remarkable natural substance that can relax muscles at the same time that it steps up reflexes. It gives you energy without resorting to the use of artificial stimulants.

You'll find soft-gel capsules with amounts from 375 mcg to 3000 mcg, or even higher. Depending on your own needs, take one capsule three times a day with meals.

Fructose

Fructose is an alternative to table sugar (sucrose), in use since 1874 for its special metabolic properties.

Fructose is sweeter than ordinary sugar and sweeter than honey. Therefore, a smaller quantity can be consumed to get the same taste.

Most people love sweets, it's one of the factors that puts weight on in the first place.

That you can use less fructose than sugar, that fructose is only partially insulin-independent, and that fructose converted into glucose will be slowly released into the bloodstream avoids the massive "insulin dump" (causing you to feel super-tired and emotionally "let down") that usually comes from the use of sugar as a sweetener. This enables those individuals with a sweet tooth, or those with sugar-related diseases to utilize fructose while minimizing the fluctuations in both high and low sugar levels that occur with table-sugar.

Cook and bake with it, replacing the sugar in your favorite recipes. Look for diet aids containing fructose, because the little bit that is present will give you an energy lift when your calorie-cutting diet tends to make you feel a little down in the mouth. Get natural fructose the way nature intended. Eat more fruit. Look for fructose-sweetened foods instead of sugary foods. You'll be amazed at the number of calories saved!

Fructose is available in health food stores and in supermarkets. Replace table sugar with a bowl of fructose, but use less of the fructose to get the same sweetness.

Vitamin B-15 (?)

B-15 is not a vitamin. Let's call it an accessory nutrient which increases both the supply of oxygen in the blood and its uptake into the body's tissues.

Dr. Robert Atkins recommends B-15 to the weary, in *Dr. Atkins' Super Energy Diet*, when none of the other vitamins work. He says that B-15 can turn a person's energy picture around surprisingly.

Natural sources include liver, seeds, rice, and whole grains. The nutrient is also available in health food stores and some drugstores. Dr. Lutz of the Institute of Preventive Medicine has recommended a dose of 50 mg to 150 mg a day. According to the FDA, B-15 is a supplement when it is used by itself and not in combination with any other substance. It does not recognize its use for any other purpose.

Guarana

Commercially available weight-reduction products contain guarana as one of the ingredients.

Guarana contains from 3 to 5 percent caffeine which is the reason for its appetite-suppressant effect.

Many diet products found in drugstores combine caffeine with propanolamine but if you are sensitive to caffeine, use caution.

It is found in 15 mg tablets or capsules in health food stores and drugstores. Follow manufacturer's instructions for use.

Herbal Fat Fighters

Many companies offer herbal combinations that have been taken from folklore.

One such contains the following: glucomannan, chickweed, burdock root, chia seed, psyllium seed and celery seed.

Because such formulas contain a large amount of fiber, they swell and expand in the stomach — providing they are taken with sufficient water.

It is said that in order to reduce the caloric density of the usual diet, you must provide extra volume to the stomach, promote the feeling of fullness and slow the rate at which calories can be ingested.

These formulas also contribute to regularity by speeding the transit time of food throughout the body. By speeding it up, mixtures such as the above help decrease the absorption of dietary cholesterol.

Along with this concept must go diet! Absolutely no junk food is to be eaten. Highly refined sugar foods throw the metabolism off and undermine all your good efforts.

Lecithin

Lecithin is found in egg yolks and in some vegetable oils, but mostly in soybean oil.

It's part of every single cell in your body and about 17 to 20 percent of the brain is made from lecithin.

Lecithin keeps your fat moving, moving right off you, and is also a natural diuretic and an effective cholesterol-reducer. In addition, it's the source of two of the hardest-to-find B-vitamins: choline and inositol. And it's loaded with sexy vitamin E.

For thousands of years (even before 1,000 B.C.), the people of China have regarded the soybean as the perfect food. One of the reasons for its reputation is that it includes all the nutritional requirements for the human diet. No other food is as rich in the protein nutrients that are needed for energy, heat, and tissue repair, and it is the only vegetable that is almost identical to the protein composition in animal food.

One major function of lecithin (also called phosphatidyl choline) is to supply choline in the diet. Choline is an important B-vitamin with the property of breaking down fat deposits that may have been on your body for twenty years.

This property is used for the treatment of atherosclerosis (fat deposits in the walls of the arteries) and other problems caused by fat accumulation.

Choline is distributed throughout our body in the blood and comes either from the food we eat, mostly as phosphatidyl choline, or from its manufacture in the liver. Our bodies do not manufacture enough choline, so we have to rely on getting it from our food or from supplements.

You can buy lecithin in granule or powder form to be mixed with food, or you can get capsules (1200 mg) or even chewable tablets with a nice vanilla taste (also 1200 mg). Try taking two capsules, or chewing two tablets, after each meal.

Crash Diets — If You Absolutely Must
Lose a Few Pounds

These diets are not intended for long-term use, but just if you have to lose from six to ten pounds in a hurry.
If you have to get into that dress or that pair of pants, try these — but not if you want to lose a lot of weight and keep it off.

Take a good vitamin and mineral formula at least twice a day, and some fiber tablets with a full glass of water before meals.

Also, in all the diets that follow (as with all food), eat vegetables and fruit at least an hour apart, because they need different enzymes in order to be digested.

Seven-Day Crash Plan

First Day

BREAKFAST:
Scrambled egg (use non-stick pan and Pam)
Whole wheat or bran muffin
Herbal tea (no sugar)

LUNCH:
Broiled hamburger on half a bun
Lettuce and tomato salad with lemon juice
Melon wedge
Herbal tea

SUPPER:
Broiled shrimp (4 ounces)
Small baked potato
Green salad with lemon juice
Small baked apple
Herbal tea

SNACK:
Apple
Club soda with lime juice

Second Day

BREAKFAST:
One medium orange
1/2 cup cooked oatmeal (sweetened with apple juice)
1/2 cup skim milk
Herbal tea

LUNCH:
1 cup clear broth
Green salad of cucumbers, beansprouts, watercress, lettuce

Cheddar cheese sandwich on whole wheat bread
Herbal tea

DINNER:
Low-salt tomato juice
Mixed salad with added green pepper
Roasted chicken without skin (3 ounces)
1 cup steamed broccoli
Herbal tea

SNACK:
1/2 cup unsweetened pineapple

Third Day

BREAKFAST:
Western omelet (use non-stick pan and Pam)
2 slices whole wheat bread (may be toasted)
Herbal tea

LUNCH:
Seafood salad of lettuce, tomatoes, and 4 broiled shrimp
Lemon-juice dressing
1 slice whole wheat bread
Herbal tea

DINNER:
Mixed green salad
Broiled sirloin steak (trimmed of fat) with sliced onions and
     mushrooms (steak to be as close to 4 ounces as possible,
     after trimming)
1/2 cup steamed carrots and peas
Angel food cake (1-inch slice)

SNACK:
1 cup fresh fruit salad

Fourth Day

BREAKFAST:
Medium orange
1 shredded wheat biscuit
1/2 cup skim milk
Herbal tea

LUNCH:
Salad of shredded apples, cabbage, carrots
Sliced turkey or chicken (without skin)
1 slice whole wheat bread (or toast)
Melon wedge
Herbal tea

DINNER:
Salad; lettuce, tomato, peppers, zucchini, lemon dressing
Broiled fillet of sole (4 ounces)
Steamed asparagus
Herbal tea

SNACK:
Fresh fruit, your choice

Fifth Day

BREAKFAST:
6 stewed prunes
Whole wheat muffin
1 pat butter
Herbal tea

LUNCH:
Lettuce and tomato salad
1 cup clear broth
Swiss cheese sandwich on whole wheat bread
Herbal tea

DINNER:
Green salad
2 small broiled lamb chops
1/2 cup steamed carrots or peas
Angel food cake (1-inch slice)
Herbal tea

SNACK:
1 cup fresh fruit salad

Sixth Day

BREAKFAST:
1/2 grapefruit
1 slice French toast
Herbal tea

LUNCH:
Mixed green salad
Tuna sandwich on whole wheat bread
Melon wedge
Herbal tea

DINNER:
Low-salt tomato juice
Mixed green salad
Broiled or roasted chicken without skin (3 ounces)
Herbal tea

SNACK:
Medium apple

Seventh Day

BREAKFAST:
1/2 cup cooked oatmeal (sweetened with apple juice)
1/2 cup skim milk

1 slice whole wheat toast with a dab of butter
Herbal tea

LUNCH:
Chef's salad of 3 ounces cubed chicken, plus cucumbers,
 lettuce, tomatoes, and radishes, with dressing of lemon
 juice or apple cider vinegar
Small baked apple
Herbal tea

DINNER:
Mixed green salad
Choice of 4 ounces salmon or swordfish
1/2 cup steamed carrots
Small baked potato
Herbal tea

SNACK:
1 cup mixed fruit

Cutting Down On Calories
Is Easier Than You Think

You don't want to jump into a 1200-calorie routine all at once.
What you really should do is take your time and lower the calorie
count week by week, losing 500 to 1,000 calories over a period of
time. In that way you will keep Diet Panic and Diet Stress under
control.

Remember to keep well-stocked with vitamins and minerals,
and keep your belly happy with fiber.

You don't have to memorize all the foods you eat with the
number of calories they contain. The group listings that follow will
give you a good approximation, and it covers most average American
choices in the diet area. For example:

BREAKFAST:
Cooked whole grain cereal
1/2 cup whole milk
1 slice whole-grain bread
Herbal tea

LUNCH:
2 ounces white meat turkey
1 cup mixed carrots and green beans
1 baked potato
Herbal tea

SUPPER:
2 hard-boiled eggs
1 slice whole-grain bread
Lettuce and tomato salad
1 cup blueberries

This menu provides a total count of only 830 calories, leaving room for reasonable snacks between meals and at bedtime.

Although this is a calorie-restricted program, it's not one that will give the average dieter too much trouble. By looking over the chart, and figuring what you like to eat and what you hate, you'll find it easy to begin to judge other foods by comparing them to the chart.

It would be difficult to eat more than 2,000 calories if you selected only from the foods shown here.

Group One — Serving Size 1 Cup — Average 35 Calories

Asparagus	Cauliflower	Lettuce
Green beans	Celery	Mushrooms
Broccoli	Cucumber	Green peppers
Cabbage	Eggplant	Radishes

Group Two — Serving Size 1 cup — average 45 calories

Artichokes	Lima beans	Peas
Bean sprouts	Rutabagas	Squash
Beets	Turnips	Baked potato
Carrots	Brussels sprouts	

Group Three — Serving size 1 cup — average 80 calories

Apple (fresh)	Cantaloupe	Plums (fresh)
Blackberries (unsweetened)	Cherries (fresh)	Strawberries (unsweetened)
Blueberries	Honeydew melon	Watermelon
Boysenberries (unsweetened)	Orange	
	Huckleberries (unsweetened)	

Group Four — Serving size as indicated — average 75 calories

Whole-grain bread (1 slice)	Granola or whole-grain dry cereal (1/2 cup)	Popcorn (1-1/2 cups)
Cooked whole-grain cereal (1/2 cup)		

Group Five — Serving size 2 ounces — average 150 calories

Beef	Eggs	Fish
Lamb	Turkey	Natural cheeses
Chicken	Liver	Cottage cheese

Group Six — Serving size as indicated — average 85 calories

Avocado (1/2)	Salad dressing (2 tbsp)	Skim milk (1 cup)
Butter (2 tsp)	Whole milk (1/2 cup)	Unflavored yogurt (1/2 cup)

If you go on any of these diets, make sure that you take a good vitamin/mineral supplement at least once a day.

Dr. Johnson's Pound-a-Week Diet

Dr. Harry Johnson, of the Life Extension Institute, tells his people not to change their diets or regular eating habits, but to cut 500 calories a day from their daily consumption.

Since 3500 calories add up to one pound of stored fat, you should lose one pound a week.

Cut your intake of bread, sugar, sweets, and desserts rather than fruits, vegetables, and meat.

The High-Protein, Low-Carbohydrate Diet

This is an eat-all-you-want diet, providing you eat certain foods.

Eat all you want of eggs, cottage cheese, meat, poultry, and fish.

Don't eat cold cuts, sausage, sugar, or starch.
Do eat two small green salads daily.
Do eat up to four ounces of cheese daily.
Don't eat any carbohydrates at all for the first ten days.

(This is not a diet you will stay on for an indefinite period of time. Just long enough to lose six to ten pounds.)

The Ultimate Diet — Fasting

For those who can tolerate total deprivation, Dr. Allan Cott and many other physicians recommend fasting as the most effective "diet" of all.

You can drink plenty of water, but no tea, coffee, or caffeine-containing drinks.

It will be difficult at first, but hunger pangs will subside after the second day or so. Weight loss will be rapid — perhaps three pounds the first day.

However, because prolonged fasting burns up muscle tissue as well as fat, never fast for more than four to seven days in a row without being under the care of a physician.

If total abstinence is too difficult, you can go on a juice and bouillon fast. Take up to eight glasses of natural or unsweetened fruit or vegetable juice, or low-calorie bouillon each day, but no solid food.

COMMENT:

People should never fast if any of these conditions is known or suspected:

Tumor	Bleeding ulcer
Cancer	Cerebral disease
Kidney disease	Gout
Liver or blood disease	Recent heart trouble
Active lung disease	Diabetes

Here is a Suggested One-Day Juice-Fast:

7:30 AM Drink the juice of one lemon mixed with 8 oz. of water
8:30   Drink a glass of fresh orange juice
9:30   Drink a glass of unsalted tomato juice
10:30   Make a cup of alfalfa tea and sip it
11:30   Drink a glass of fresh apple juice
12:30 PM Drink eight ounces of water
1:30   Drink a glass of grape juice
4:30   Drink a glass of pineapple juice
5:30   Drink a glass of prune juice
6:30   Make a cup of peppermint tea and sip it
7:30   Drink a glass of grapefruit juice
8:30   Make a cup of chamomile tea and sip it
9:30   Go to bed

Briefly here are a few of the nutritional values you've had during your juice-fast:

9 gm protein
195 mg calcium
2620 IU vitamin A
365 mg vitamin C
35 mg B-complex
Don't get on the scales until the next morning!

Nibble Diet

Put together on the table:
1 hard boiled egg
1/2 pound of sliced tomatoes
1/2 cup cottage cheese
2 thin slices of ham
1/2 ounce of hard cheese
1/4 pound of grapes
Then divide all the food into six portions. This is all you will be allowed to eat.

Seven-day Grapefruit Diet

Get your self-control ready. You can lose up to five pounds in five days. You must have grapefruit before every meal.

Don't weigh yourself every day. Step on the scales the day before your diet begins; then stay off for the next seven days. Weigh yourself on the eighth day.

Don't eat any fruit, except grapefruit and lemon.
Don't eat any milk, cheese, or cream.
Don't have any sauces thickened with flour or eggs.
Don't use chili sauce, ketchup, or mayonnaise.
Don't eat corn or beets.
Don't eat pudding, rice, potatoes, bread, or pasta.
Don't use any sugar.

This is your menu for the next seven days:

BREAKFAST:
1/2 grapefruit
Meat or fish prepared any way you like it, as long as it is not made with a sauce
Green or raw-vegetable salad with apple cider vinegar or lemon juice dressing
Herb tea with lemon, or black coffee

DINNER:
1/2 grapefruit
Meat or fish cooked the way you like best, but no sauce
Green or yellow vegetable
Tea or black coffee

BEDTIME:
4 ounces unsweetened grapefruit juice

Make sure you are taking a strong vitamin and mineral tablet morning and night to provide any missing nutrients. You'll notice there are no suggested portions of either fish or meat. That's because you can have a good portion of either just as long as it is baked or broiled, grilled or even sauteed, but without any sauce when served.

This is not a diet you should stay on for any length of time. Seven to ten days ought to get you into that dream dress.

Sea-Vegetable Diet

For those who would like the weight-loss benefits of sea vegetables, but who do not want to take kelp tablets, the following recipes should be interesting.Try using one of these dishes once daily. The ingredients are available from your supermarket or from your local health food store.

Sea-Vegetable Rolls:
    3 avocados
    1/2 cabbage, chopped finely
    2 cups alfalfa sprouts
    2 tbsp lemon juice
    1 package nori sheets

Mash avocados and mix in cabbage, sprouts, and lemon juice.
Cut nori sheets in half.
Spread mixture on sheets, roll and serve.

Wakame and Cabbage Salad:
    2 cups cabbage sprouts
    2 cups cabbage, finely chopped
    1/2 cup wakame, soaked for 15 minutes and then drained.

Mix well together and serve with sesame dressing.

Sesame Dressing:
Soak 1 cup sesame seeds in a jar overnight.
Pour off the water and rinse well, then add a little water to make a
paste.
Pour over the salad and add your favorite vegetables if desired.

Sea Guacamole:
    2 avocados
    2 tbsp. lemon juice
    1 stalk celery, chopped
    1 scallion
    1 cup radish sprouts
    1/2 cup dry dulse in small pieces

Mash avocados and mix well with the lemon juice.
Add vegetables and dulse. Mix well and serve.

Sea-Vegetable Salad:
    1 cup arame
    1 cup dulse
    3 scallions
    2 red peppers
    4 mushrooms
    1 small clove garlic
    1/2 cup lemon juice

Soak arame for about ten minutes and then drain.
Rinse dulse three times and mix with the arame.
Dice peppers, mushrooms, and scallions. Mix together.
Mix garlic and lemon juice in a blender and pour over the sea
vegetables.
Mix well.

Contraindications

Before you go on any diet, make sure you can go on a diet
without causing some problems. For most of us this means going to
the doctor for a checkup.

Also, although the substances mentioned in this chapter are all
natural and available without a prescription, there are some cautions
to be observed.

Arginine and Ornithine

These are not to be used by people suffering from diabetes,
ocular or brain herpes infection, pituitary dysfunction, or cancer.

GTF Chromium

Not to be used if you are allergic to yeast.

Fiber

Large amounts can interfere with absorption of nutrients from the food you eat. When using fiber, be sure you take supplemental vitamins and minerals.

L-Carnitine

The use of D-carnitine or D-L carnitine has been associated with several severe side effects. Make sure that the substance you are using is pure L-carnitine.

L-Phenylalanine

Do not use this supplement if you are taking a MAO inhibitor (some antidepressants). If you are not sure, ask your physician.

Do not use if you have cardiac arrhythmias, hypertension (high blood pressure), the genetic disease PKU, psychosis, or existing pigmented malignant melanoma type cancer, or if you have a violent temper.

Caution: if you are severely depressed, do not attempt to treat yourself, but do see a physician! There are many causes of depression, and your problem must be understood and dealt with accordingly.

L-Tryptophan

Some individuals may be stimulated by the use of this amino acid instead of relaxed. Such individuals should not continue its use, since it is not readily apparent why this side effect occurs.

As this is going to press, the FDA is temporarily recommending a maximum dosage of 100 mg daily.

L-Tyrosine

If you have a history of high blood pressure, you should monitor your pressure when using L-tyrosine. Do not use L-tyrosine if you use MAO inhibitors, have cardiac arrhythmias, psychosis, preexisting malignant melanoma-type cancer, or if you have a violent temper.

Kelp

This should not be used to treat yourself for an underactive or overactive thyroid condition without the consent of your physician.

What is Obesity?

Scientists consider obesity to be 20 percent or more over the ideal weight. The tables below are based on the ones used by Metropolitan Life for ages 25 to 59. The third figure in the column shows the approximate threshold of obesity.

MEN

HEIGHT	SMALL		MEDIUM		LARGE	
5' 2"	125-131	157	128-138	166	135-148	178
5' 3"	127-133	160	130-140	168	137-151	181
5' 4"	129-135	162	132-143	172	139-155	186
5' 5"	131-137	164	134-146	175	141-159	191
5' 6"	133-140	168	137-149	179	144-163	196
5' 7"	135-143	172	140-152	182	147-167	200
5' 8"	137-146	175	143-155	186	150-171	205
5' 9"	139-149	179	146-158	190	153-175	210
5'10"	141-152	182	149-161	193	156-179	215
5'11"	144-155	186	152-165	198	159-183	220
6' 0"	147-159	191	155-169	203	163-187	224
6' 1"	150-163	196	159-173	208	167-192	230
6' 2"	153-167	200	162-177	212	171-197	236
6' 3"	157-171	205	166-182	218	176-202	242

WOMEN

HEIGHT	SMALL		MEDIUM		LARGE	
4' 9"	99-108	130	106-118	142	115-128	154
4'10"	100-110	132	108-120	144	117-131	157
4'11"	101-112	134	110-123	148	119-134	161
5' 0"	103-115	138	112-126	151	122-137	164
5' 1"	105-118	142	115-129	155	125-140	168
5' 2"	108-121	145	118-132	158	128-144	173
5' 3"	111-124	149	121-135	162	131-148	178
5' 4"	114-127	152	124-138	166	134-152	172
5' 5"	117-130	156	127-141	169	137-156	187
5' 6"	120-133	160	130-144	173	140-160	192
5' 7"	123-136	163	133-147	176	143-164	197
5' 8"	126-139	167	136-150	180	146-167	200
5' 9"	129-142	170	139-153	184	149-170	204
5'10"	132-145	174	142-156	187	152-173	208

The Seven Day

Super Potency Diet

The Instant Virility Diet for
Men & Women of All Ages

by Dr. William H. Lee

Foreplay

Sex begins in the mind, then spreads down to the genitals.

The mind is contiguous with the brain.

The brain needs good food to precipitate good sex.

Good sex needs the staple foods of a sexually healthly culture to manufacture the brain chemicals necessary to stimulate the pleasure-making neural pathways all the way down to the biochemical impulses of orgasm.

Sexual arousal is more than me Tarzan, you Jane.

Sexual arousal is time and place, biochemistry, hormones, nutrients, energizers, stimulants, antioxidants, mood elevators, and two people.

Are there aphrodisiacs?

Yes, and chief among them is your diet. Certain foods are capable of supplying the body with the nutritional elements to support sexual arousal. Other foods simply make you sleepy!

But there's more.

We've also learned how to trick the brain into manufacturing the brain chemicals that are more conducive to lovemaking. And these can actually stimulate the "old" brain, the brain that was so active during the cave days when sex was more important than eating because the race had to survive.

Nature built in a powerful sex drive that unleashed provocative, stimulating neurotransmitters which had to be satisfied, and not only one time!

When you begin to practice diet and nutritional control, results begin in the first month and build slowly as your body starts to appreciate the raw material and supplemental nutritional income. Don't rush things. As nature begins to intervene let the fullness slowly improve everything you do . . .

In these modern times when casual sex has become a threat, the old adage of treating a wife like a mistress and a husband like a "john," makes a lot more sense.

Variety is no longer the spice of life, but that doesn't mean that sexual pleasure has to be forgotten. It only means that innovation and stimulation are needed to get the glands working. Slippery, sliding, sticky foods can do a lot. Try some of these "whored'oeuvres" before your next encounter!

Honey

Don't keep the bottle in the fridge.

Honey should be warm, wet, sticky sweet like your first night . . . the honeymoon.

Honey is made from flower nectar, incubated in the stomach of a bee, predigested into the fructose food energy that can stimulate desire. Fructose is also part of the male semen. It provides energy to the whipping tails of the sperm on their mad route to mate with an egg.

Fructose is instantly converted to sexual energy and burned for body energy without the need for wasteful digestion. It goes straight to the male organ where it's needed. It's the easiest, fastest source of renewed male potency.

In Morocco, as in many other lands, a wedding celebration prepares the couples for conjugal bliss by providing honey cakes to be eaten with a drink of honey ale.

This combination lends itself to super-fast replenishment of semen for another go around . . .

The *Perfumed Garden* adds to the precoital meal and insures satisfaction with twenty almonds and 100 pine nuts. Not so farfetched! Almonds contain protein, linoleic acid, iron, calcium, potassium, vitamins B-1, B-2, B-3, and contains a huge charge of erection-stimulating phosphorus.

Pine nuts are no slouch in the nutrition department. They contain quantities of protein, calcium, potassium, B-1, B-2, B-3, and another batch of phosphorus.

Put them together with honey for energy and aspartic acid (stamina when you need it), the B-Complex vitamins, potassium, sulfur, calcium, sodium, phosphorus, magnesium, silicon, iron, manganese and copper, and you can see why the author of the *Perfumed Garden* knew what he was talking about.

What is amazing is that it was written in the 1600's before anybody understood the basis of sexual energy!

We're not only talking to men.

Women athletes lick a teaspoonful of honey before competing so they can get that extra "push."

Honey helps calcium absorption and helps to improve the oxygen content of the blood. And that extra oxygen means more energy for the sex act, freer movement, plus explosive new enjoyment.

Stick your fingers in honey and have your partner slowly lick the honey from them. Or anywhere else for that matter. This kind of enjoyment may sound "kinky" to some people until they try it for the first time, then they're sold.

Honey is not a lubricant.

Honey is an anti-lubricant.

If age has interfered with some of the enjoyment with less elasticity and less joyful tight contact, consider this ability. Think of its sensation-increasing role in mouth to organ contact.

Honey is a natural, inexpensive, and often startling aphrodisiac for use with free-wheeling abandon by both partners.

Lecithin and Phos-Chol

There's the old story about the aging man who went to the doctor complaining that he keeps chasing his young secretary around the room.

"What's wrong with that?" asked the doctor.

The man replied, "When I catch her I forget why I was chasing her in the first place."

Not so funny in the light of what we know today. Certain brain chemicals help us to remember things. The main one is called acetylcholine and it's manufactured from choline we get in the diet. If there's not enough from foods, we can supplement the amount with lecithin. Two 1200 milligram capsules with each meal can help.

There's a stronger version called Phos-Chol which is about 85% pure choline. One or two capsules with meals will help the production of this important neurotransmitter which has a lot to do with sexual arousal and feeling. When taking the supplement, take about 50 milligrams of pantothenic acid to help it along.

Lecithin also contributes to the production of adrenal hormones which are essential to sexual excitement. It also helps the circulation. Since sexual stimulation depends on blood suffusing the sex organs, male and female, a free-flowing bloodstream is conducive to increased desire and orgasm.

Lecithin is a rich source of phosphorus, one of the sexiest minerals around.

Add it to your nutritional regimen.

Bee Pollen

Ounce for ounce it is a better protein than meat or eggs, and the amino acid content is better than any other food. It contains all 22 of the known elements that comprise the human body.

Bee pollen, sometimes called bee bread, contains a hormone that is almost an exact copy of human sex hormone, gonadotropin. The ancient desert Bedouins somehow knew of this and used it to master their harems.

Nutrition-oriented physicians now suggest it for greater sexual endurance. The natural enzymes, amino acids, hormones, vitamins and minerals appear to nourish the neurogenital reflex.

Sprinkle pollen on your breakfast cereal, or on cottage cheese, apple sauce or your yogurt for better and longer lasting sexual functioning.

Royal Jelly

It's what makes a queen from an ordinary bee beginning. Somehow, this thin, milky fluid has the power to transform any immature bee into a queen. What's its secret? Nobody knows for sure but it's loaded with protein, vitamins and particularly pantothenic acid with a special enzyme that makes this powerful vitamin easier to absorb.

We know that pantothenic acid is essential to the adrenal glands. Along with vitamin C, the two nutrients help to fuel this most important energy source. This helps the body combat numbing daily stress — with more than enough reserve for nightly sex.

Royal jelly is available in capsule form, not only for the queen among humans but also for the king.

Milk

Milk is one of the best sources of calcium, especially when the milk is fortified with vitamin D to help with the assimilation of the calcium.

In the *Kama Sutra* of Vatsyayana (Burton Version):

The fastest means of increasing sexual vigor by food and drink are as follows:

1) A man obtains sexual vigor by drinking milk mixed with sugar, the piper chaba (pepper), and licorice.

2) Drinking milk with sugar and the boiled testicle of a ram or goat.

3) Taking the husks of the sesame seeds, soaking them with the eggs of the sparrow (hens' eggs are just as good), boiling them with milk mixed with sugar and ghee (clarified butter) and the flour of wheat and beans. (This formula was originally intended for use at an orgy with many sexual contacts in a single night.)

4) Mixing ghee, honey, sugar and licorice in equal quantities, and adding the juice of the fennel plant and milk. This composition is sweet like nectar and is said to be provocative of sexual vigor.

In the *Perfumed Garden*, Shakykh Nafzawi drank camel's milk well fortified with honey as a restorative for love's labors.

Cow's milk contains zinc. The male genitalia utilizes zinc in large amounts for seminal production. Is there a connection between ancient and modern knowledge? You bet there is . . .

The Law of Similars

Oysters look like testicles.
The ancient peoples believed in the law of similars.

If something resembled a part of the body, it was put there by nature to treat that part of the body. So, oysters were good for the testicles and would increase sexual congress and fertility.

Turns out that they're right. Not because they look like testicles but because they contain the nutrients that testicles need to stay healthy.

A whole branch of medicine sprang up based on the law of similars. If a plant grew in the water it was good for the genito-urinary system. If it grew in the air and the ground, the part that was in the air was good for the head and lungs while the part that grew underground was meant for the parts of the body from the waist down.

Nuts

Nuts are for nuts!

Nuts are plant seeds. They are close to 50% polyunsaturated oil. They are excellent sources of the nutrients needed to manufacture the primitive sex hormones. They turn your body into a vast laboratory for manufacturing the sex hormones you've dreamed about for years. They are also great sources of vitamins E, B-Complex, phosphorus, magnesium, potassium, manganese, vanadium, molybdenum and fabulous zinc.

Zinc is now being accepted by the medical profession as one of the prime minerals for sexual renewal.

Nuts, milk, seafood, liver and whole wheat contain this very needed mineral.

Eat nuts raw. Add them to a green salad. Grind them with bananas and milk with a dash of honey for the 'ready-to-go' pickup you need after a full day at work.

From the Sea

We came from the sea.

The sea contains many elements we need to sustain life and love.

Why do so many people revere caviar? It's only fish eggs, the roe from sturgeons. Why is it tops in the sex game?

In every 100 grams of roe there is 335 milligrams of bio-active phosphorus. Fresh, organic, been-through-the-fish's-body, ready-for-active-use phosphorus!

In ancient Egypt, they were so sexually stimulating that they were banned to the priesthood.

Caviar is the treatment of choice in nutritionally reversible impotence. Because it contains vast amounts of the basic mineral needed for repeated muscle contraction, it contributes happily to orgasm after orgasm.

Your diet should include eels, shellfish (clams, oysters, mussels, shrimps and crabs). Seafood is a source of iodine and iodine is needed by the thyroid gland. The thyroid gland regulates your basal metabolism, the rate at which your body normally works. If the gland is sluggish you will have little need or desire for sex.

If you can't afford good caviar, buy second-rate caviar. If that is also out of your reach, here's a recipe so powerful that she may just keep you in bed all weekend long:

    1 tablespoon of anchovy paste
    1 tablespoon minced chives
    1 tablespoon chopped pimento
    1/2 teaspoon lemon juice
    Spread on thin toast and feed both of you.

Got a guy who just won't make the first step? Make him a special tuna salad:

    1 can of tuna
    sliced cucumbers
    lettuce
    radishes
    tomatoes
    Spanish capers
    grated raw carrots
    drop of mayonnaise

Or, try an oyster salad:

1 dozen oysters, shucked
lettuce
cooked and sliced beetroot
olives
tomatoes
grated raw carrots
onions or leeks
lemon juice
salt and pepper to taste

Arrange all of the ingredients on a platter and feed each other.
Sounds simple and it is . . . but you'll be thrilled with the results.

Sea Soup

You'll have to go to the health food store to buy some of these
products. Ask for Dulse, Irish moss or Nori. They are seaweeds to
be made into soup or sometimes added to salads. Seaweeds are rich
in iodine (the thyroid-fueling element) as well as vanadium,
chromium, bromine, lithium and vitamins A, B-Complex, C, D, and K.
The packages have instructions on how to use the seaweeds
and although the taste will be a bit foreign to you, you'll soon get
used to it and look for the lift you get after a bowl of seaweed soup.

Salad Bar is No Bar to Sex

Find a place that steams vegetables and feed your sex.
Don't cook vegetables until they're limp. It gives your body
the wrong idea. Raw or lightly steamed only.

Asparagus

Was a medicine before it became a food. Loaded with
vitamins A, B-Complex, C, manganese, iron, phosphorus and rutin.
The "cat pee" odor it gives to the urine is from asparagine — a great

source of comfort to the genito-urinary system. Rutin with vitamin C helps strengthen capillaries, those essential tiny blood vessels that deliver blood to the sex organ.

Culpepper, the herbalist, claimed that a brew of asparagus roots boiled in wine and taken early in the morning for several days running "stirreth up bodily lust in man or woman."

The *Perfumed Garden* agrees with Culpepper but says that the asparagus stalk should be blanched and sauteed. Although noted Parisian Josephine Baker swore by another stiff fruit — the banana — most Parisians follow Rabelais's "uniterminal, intercrural asparagus stalk."

Avocado

Powerful source of protein, vitamins A, E, B-Complex plus 17 minerals and amino acids.

It is a virtually complete food and easily digested. It brings vitamin A to you in the form of Beta-carotene, a disease fighter and fatigue fighter.

Its amino acid content helps to build neurotransmitters which, in turn, stimulate sexual activity.

It even helps fight bacterial invaders of the urinary tract by making the area more acidic.

Eat them when you find them. You can make an avocado salad by mashing the soft pulp with some apple cider vinegar and safflower oil and mixing in lettuce, tomatoes, raw onion and radishes.

With some whole wheat toast and one glass of wine (one glass only), both of you will be set for an enjoyable romp in the hay!

Bananas

Firm, stiff and delicious when ready.

Bananas provide vitamins A, B-Complex, C, E, potassium and other minerals.

They help to stabilize nerve functions and increase your sexual energy.

Green Beans

Help stimulate kidney function and liver function and contain vitamins A, B-Complex, C, inositol, phosphorus, calcium, copper, cobalt and chlorophyll.

If you don't like them as a vegetable then put them through your juicer and combine the juice with some carrot juice every day. It helps ward off joint pains.

Carrots

They need a book alone. Carrots contain vitamins A, Beta-carotene, B-complex, C, iron, phosphorus, calcium, sodium, potassium, magnesium, manganese, sulfur, copper, bromine, asparagine, and a substance called daucarine.

A healthy body is a sexy body and carrots will help you get and stay healthy. Daucarine is a strong blood vessel dilator and may be of erectile help.

Garlic & Onions

As long as you both eat them . . .

In early Rome, they were used as a "cure" for an "exhausted penis."

Petronious recommended snails and onions as a sexual stimulant for both sexes.

The *Perfumed Garden* tells of the hero having to satisfy a number of women in a row, fortifying his loins with a drink of honey and onion juice.

Garlic helps lower blood pressure, fight infections, lower cholesterol and rid the body of unwanted chemicals.

Food Parts to "Trick" the Body

Do you know that you can trick your body into thinking you're sexually up to 30 years younger?

You can do it with stimulating foods (protein makes you more active and carbohydrates make you less active) or, you can go to the active ingredients in certain foods — take them in supplement form — and *actually have the body make those chemicals that make you more sexy!*

Essentially those food parts are amino acids that you can buy in health food stores or drug stores.

If you know which foods to use when, you can stimulate your erotic areas at will, or calm them down again.

You can improve your sex life.

You can improve your mood.

You can tip the erectal dice in your favor so you no longer have to depend on chance.

Why use supplements to get food parts?

Why not just eat the foods?

Here's the reason . . . the food parts have to reach the brain. If you eat food, the parts needed to influence the brain travel through the bloodstream to the brain in more-or-less equal amounts. They pass the blood-brain barrier together and normal feelings occur.

What you want is to command your brain to make excessive quantities of sex hormones. In order to do that, you need certain food parts to be available in greater concentration than if they were found in the foods that naturally carry them.

Norepinephrine is one of the brain chemicals that is important to memory and learning. It is also important to primitive drives such as sex!

Without enough norepinephrine people tend to become depressed and depressed people don't incline toward sexual pleasure.

Two food parts (amino acids) called L-phenylalanine and L-tyrosine help the brain manufacture norepinephrine. So, if you take either of them between meals or before bedtime — with a tablet or capsule of the B-Complex vitamins — you start to tilt your feelings in favor of sex.

Both of these amino acids are found in eggs, meat, chicken, and cheese, but it's easier to get a larger amount into the brain if you take a supplement.

Eat the sex foods as part of your menu and try the supplements for an added jolt.

Depending on the person, an effective dose can be from 100 milligrams to 500 milligrams.

There is one caution connected to the use of L-phenylalanine. It can raise blood pressure in some individuals. In that case, with your doctor's consent, try the L-tyrosine instead.

(ALSO — L-phenylalanine should not be used if phenylketonuria (PKU) is present or if there is a pigmented melanoma.)

(FINALLY — in all cases, during pregnancy or lactation, nothing that is not recommended by a doctor should be used.)

We all know that an anxious lover is a lousy lover!

If the idea of actually being able to manipulate the manufacture of brain chemicals to influence moods is intriguing to you, imagine being able to calm anxiety.

The brain chemical in this case is called serotonin and the amino acid which exerts influence is called L-tryptophan. Potatoes and pasta, fish and peanuts, meat and dairy products contain this amino acid. But, to exert influence you need the supplement. Take one tablet before sex to drain away anxiety. Just one because two of them might help you to be so calm that you'll fall asleep.

A bite or two of a banana and a tablet of L-tryptophan and happy sex and a good night's sleep . . .

(ONE LAST CAUTION — if you're taking monamine oxidase inhibitors [MAO I], don't take any amino acid supplements.)

Vitamin/Mineral Nutrition and Sex

Good sex needs good food.

Good food supplies all the nutrients needed by the body.

Good food supplies all the vitamins, minerals and trace elements critical to normal sex drive.

All nutrients are needed but some are more important to your sexual life than others. If it's not in your diet or you suspect you're not getting enough . . . take supplements!

Here's some of the needed nutrients and why:

We can't make vitamins and minerals except in very rare instances. We have to get them from food or supplements.

Vitamin A

A deficiency of this vitamin results in the atrophy of testicles in the male rat and ovaries in a female rat and also in loss of sperm production, reabsorption of the fetus and more horrible situations. Nobody should be low in vitamin A when it's so easy to obtain. (Found in fish, fish liver oil, liver, eggs, cheese, yogurt, green leafy vegetables, fruits, etc.)

Vitamin A protects the mucous membrane of the vagina, keeping it young, smooth, soft and lubricated. It makes skin lovely to touch and helps to ward off bacterial invasion.

The B-Complex Family of Vitamins

These vitamins are essential to energy production. Try having sex without the energy to carry it through. The B-vitamins are necessary for the metabolism of all the protein, carbohydrates and fats you eat.

A riboflavin (B-2) deficiency robs you of energy very quickly since it is deeply involved in your energy-producing cycles.

Niacin (B-3) can affect your sex life through your nerves or your digestive tract when it is deficient. However, niacin has the ability to *gorge sexual arteries with blood and stimulate circulation to the extremities*. When you consider extremities, one end is the brain and the other is your . . . other end!

Good food sources are lean meat, chicken, fish, asparagus, dates, almonds, yogurt and raw seeds. Niacin should be in your multi-vitamin.

Pyridoxine (vitamin B-6) is involved in the health of your nerves and is important in the manufacture of brain chemicals. It helps to make norepinephrine, one of the sex neurotransmitters, in the brain. Lack of vitamin B-6 in the pituitary glands can result in a loss of the sex drive.

B-6 is found in wheat germ and wheat bran, raw nuts and seeds, honey and molasses.

Pantothenic acid is needed for energy production and helps in the manufacture of steroid hormones and the neurotransmitters necessary for sexual arousal.

Try liver, milk, eggs, whole grains, raw nuts and seeds, broccoli and cabbage.

Biotin, PABA, Folic Acid, Choline, Inositol, and vitamin B-12 are all part of the B-Complex and should be included in any supplemental regimin.

Choline is necessary to sexual arousal.

Inositol is considerd to be the "youth" vitamin. Both choline and inositol are found in lecithin. Lecithin is needed by both the brain and the sexual system.

Folic acid deficiency can cause spontaneous abortion.

B-12 deficiency will reduce the desire for sex.

Vitamin C

Has a direct effect on the sexual system through its role in iron absorption which affects hemoglobin and energy, and its role with the health of the adrenal glands. The adrenal gland stores great quantities of vitamin C but needs replenishing every day. It is the adrenal gland which makes several hormones and neurotransmitters *including the hormone involved in stimulating orgasm.*

Best food sources are strawberries, tomatoes, mangoes, brussel sprouts, avocados, and citrus fruits.

Vitamin D

If there is insufficient vitamin D in the diet, calcium absorption will be limited. Because the calcium-to-phosphorus ratio must be held constant in the body, when there is less calcium absorbed, the body eliminates phosphorus. Phosphorus is a very important mineral to the entire sexual arousal system. This is why the nutritional approach to sex is so important. All nutrients are involved and the lack of one nutrient important to your sexual health can wreak havoc on everything you do or don't do in bed!

Vitamin E

You can't spell SEX without the "E".

The hormones of the pituitary and adrenal glands are protected from destruction in the body by vitamin E and its companion selenium.

Vitamin E also increases erotic muscle recovery — giving you that "I can go on and on" feeling.

Vitamin E does many other beneficial things in the body but this chapter is primarily devoted to sex.

Vitamin F

Although there is no such thing as vitamin F, it does stand for essential fatty acids. These substances (linoleic acid, linolenic acid, arachiodonica acid) found in vegetable oils such as safflower oil, sunflower oil, olive oil and other unsaturated oils and mono-saturated oils, are needed by the body to manufacture prostaglandins (hormone-like substances which govern the second-by-second activities). They are necessary to the thyroid gland, adrenal glands, prostate gland and other body parts as well.

Max EPA (from fish) and GLA (gamma linolenic acid) can be found in health food and drugstores in capsule form. You can take Max EPA or GLA three times a day with meals.

Diet sources of vitamin F include raw nuts and seeds, whole grains, wheat germ and milk.

Minerals

Calcium

Everyone knows calcium is needed for strong bones and strong teeth. Few know that calcium affects the production of hormones by the endocrine glands, affects the menstrual cycle, and affects the sexual functioning of both men and women.

A calcium deficiency can reduce both the interest in sex and the ability to carry out the sex act.

Silicon

Although you have heard much about silicon and its use in chips . . . Silicon Valley in California, etc., you probably don't know that it is an essential mineral needed by the body for a variety of jobs.

Without silicon, your hair, nails and skin would lack the appearance, feel and beauty of health.

But more importantly to this chapter, an *enjoyable sex life would be impossible without this mineral* since silicon helps to manufacture the nerve coverings that thrill and delight us.

Silicon is found in sprouts, brown rice, whole grains, some forms of lettuce . . . but it's easier to get in the health food store in capsules. One a day should do it.

Potassium

This mineral is needed for healthy nerves and muscles. Without a sufficient amount in your body, you would be too uncoordinated to carry out the sex act.

In the diet, eat dried fruits, bananas, raw nuts and seeds, lima beans, brown rice, avocados and lean meat.

Iron

A deficiency in this mineral can cause anemia with its terrible fatigue and loss of interest in sex.

Most of the iron in your food is not absorbed. To increase the availability, vitamin C should be taken at the same time you eat iron-rich foods.

Try liver, eggs, green leafy vegetables, almonds, asparagus, fish, poultry, prunes, raisins and apricots.

Sulfur

Hard to find in supplement form but some stores have it. Sulfur is a body cleanser and helps keep the sex line open and free from impurities. Sulfur is a youth mineral. You'll find sulfur in onions, garlic, leeks, cauliflower, broccoli, brussel sprouts, asparagus, eggs, cabbage, kale, figs, parsnips, and turnips. All those "smelly" foods that are so good for us.

Phosphorus

This is the element essential to nerves, brain action, and human sexuality. *No phosphorus . . . no sex life!*

Lecithin is phosphorus, acetylcholine is phosphorus, choline is phosphorus . . . all essential for sex.

The best sources are eggs, fish eggs, seafood. Less important sources are seeds and nuts when raw (heat destroys most of the nutrient value), whole grains, brown rice, legumes, cabbage, corn and some other vegetables.

Lecithin, choline tablets, Phos-Chol, and other supplements are available at health food and drugstores.

Iodine

The thyroid gland is called the "emotional" gland. It needs iodine to manufacture the essential chemical element thyroxine. Thyroxine controls the body's production and utilization of energy.

An underactive thyroid can result in a loss of sex drive. Try dulse, kelp, pineapple, and, if you have to use salt, use iodized salt.

Magnesium

Magnesium is a relaxant as calcium is a contractant. We need to relax to enjoy lovemaking because too much stress will inhibit the joyful atmosphere. Magnesium lowers anxiety and improves performance.

It is found in leafy green vegetables, cornmeal, raw nuts and seeds, wheat germ, whole grains, seafood, dulse, legumes and milk.

Manganese, needed in many enzyme reactions, is essential to human sexuality. If you don't have it — you just don't have sex! It is found in whole grains, green vegetables, eggs, raw nuts and seeds, pineapples, apples and apricots.

Chromium helps to regulate the blood sugar level which determines energy availability.

Germanium is a new discovery which alleviates mood disorders associated with the lack of a sex drive. Found in garlic, ginseng and some leafy green vegetables. Also found as a supplement that can be purchased in health food stores.

Selenium works wonders with vitamin E.

Zinc is needed for the proper maintenance of the male and the female sexual system. A zinc deficiency may be related to a loss of sexual interest. Try oysters, fish roe, eggs, wholegrain cereals, raw nuts and seeds.

First Week — Exotic Beginning 7 Day
Sex-Stimulating Diet

This begins your new super-potent self. After the first week you can pick and choose from the menus which follow. But for the first seven days, follow every step of this regime precisely:

MONDAY
Orange juice
Scrambled eggs with fried onions
Yogurt sprinkled with fresh wheat germ
Milk, whole or skim

Pineapple juice
Cottage cheese and 1/2 grapefruit
Violet leaf tea with honey and lemon juice

Apple juice
Broiled fish with garlic sauce
Brown rice
Broccoli, steamed
Mint tea with honey and lemon juice

ALL DAYS
One multi-vitamin mineral tablet or capsule with breakfast and supper.
Other supplements to be taken as needed for your particular lifestyle.
Two lecithin capsules (1200 mg each) with meals, 1 deodorized garlic
capsule with meals, Royal jelly and other supplements as needed.

TUESDAY
Carrot juice
Oatmeal sprinkled with wheat germ and milk and honey
Whole grain toast with a smear of peanut butter
Milk

Prune juice
Hot bean soup
Steamed vegetables topped with walnuts
Yogurt and bananas
Whole grain crackers
Rose hips tea with lemon and honey

Celery and carrot juice
Liver and onions
Baked potato with yogurt
Tossed fresh salad
Fresh fruit cup
Oatstraw tea with honey and lemon

Appropriate supplements

WEDNESDAY
Grapefruit juice
Cheese omelet with fried onions or sprinkled with
    garlic powder
Bran muffins
Milk
Raspberry juice
Vegetable soup
Salmon salad with raw onion
Orange and grapefruit mix
Mixed nuts
Lemon verbena tea with honey and lemon

Fig juice
Pot roast
Tossed fresh green salad
Bread pudding
Lavender flower tea with honey and lemon

Appropriate supplements

THURSDAY
Apricot juice
Oatmeal and bran
Wholegrain toast with almond butter
Hard-boiled egg
Milk

Pomegranate juice
Beansprouts, cheddar cheese, onion,
    tomato sandwich on whole wheat bread
Coleslaw
Nuts and apricots
Watercress tea with honey and lemon
Cranberry juice
Baked chicken with snow peas
Brown rice

Pickled cabbage
Nuts and tangerines
Linden flower tea with honey and lemon

Appropriate supplements

FRIDAY
Guava juice
Bran and granola
Poached egg on whole wheat toast
Cottage cheese
Fenugreek tea

Apricot juice
Clam chowder
Grilled cheese sandwich on whole wheat
Radish and celery salad
Applesauce rosemary tea with honey and lemon

Black cherry juice
Meatloaf
Baked sweet potatoes
Peas and carrots
Coleslaw with green grapes
Strawberry tea with honey and lemon

Appropriate supplements

SATURDAY
Carrot juice
Oatmeal with dried fruit, wheat germ
Bran muffin
Milk

Strawberry juice
Sardines with raw onions

Carrot strips, radishes, lettuce, bananas,
    sunflower seeds
Alfalfa tea with honey and lemon

Orange juice
Beef stew
Fresh green salad
Yogurt sprinkled with wheat germ
Violet leaf tea with honey and lemon

Appropriate supplements

SUNDAY
Grapefruit juice
Bacon and eggs (take an extra vitamin C tablet)
Whole-wheat toast
Yogurt with wheat germ
Pineapple juice
Braised liver with onions
Fresh fruit salad
Orange flower tea with honey and lemon

Grape juice
Tuna fish with lemon juice
Wholegrain noodles, peas
Fresh tossed salad
Linden flower tea with honey and lemon

Sex-Nutrition Meal Planner — For Every
Breakfast, Lunch, and Dinner

Mix & Match from these examples to fuel a flagging sexual drive:

BREAKFASTS
Muesli with dried fruit
Hard-boiled egg
Wholegrain toast

Milk
Millet cereal
Bananas and dates
Eggs, cheese or nut butter, if desired
Milk

Fresh pineapple slices with shredded coconut
Buckwheat cereal
Baked apple
Applesauce and raisins
Canteloupe and strawberries
Toast

Fresh figs with oatmeal
Toast with nut butter
Applesauce
Milk

Prunes
Brown rice with cinnamon and raisins
Grapefruit
Poached eggs, if desired
Milk

Rice bran cereal
Dried fruit
Scrambled eggs
Wholegrain toast
Milk

Melon balls
Edam cheese on toast
Milk

LUNCHES
Tuna salad and sprouts
Pita bread

Apple and raisin salad
Oatstraw tea

Nut butter on wholegrain bread
Fresh green salad with raw onion
Fresh fruit salad
Herb tea

Carrot and cashew salad
Steamed broccoli
Brown rice
Vegetable soup

Cream of celery soup
Steamed barley
Fresh green salad with lemon and apple cider vinegar
Tea

Sardines with raw onion on a bed of lettuce
Baked yams and turnip greens
Catnip tea

Steamed vegetable salad
Lima beans
Baked potato with yogurt
Spearmint tea

Raw vegetables with lemon juice
Steamed asparagus
Brown rice and bananas
Herbal tea

Fresh green salad
Baked green pepper, eggplant and tomato stuffing
Potatoes and yogurt
Herbal tea

Salmon steak
Baked zucchini with okra
Fresh green salad
Carrot soup

DINNERS
Omelet
Vegetable broth
Steamed spinach with diced carrots and celery
Whole-grain bread
Herbal tea

Broiled fish
Fresh green salad
Cauliflower and beets
Catnip tea

Cottage cheese
Apples, peaches, grapes and raw nuts
Apple concentrate juice
Poached fresh salmon
Fresh green salad
Baked eggplant with swiss chard
Herbal tea

Tofu with soy sauce
Leek soup with added mixed green
Fresh green salad with olive oil and apple
    cider vinegar

Clams Casino
Diced carrots and steamed peas
Tomato aspic
Lamb (roast leg)
Herbal tea

Gazpacho soup
Spinach, mushrooms, 1 hard-boiled egg,
    2 slices of bacon,
1/2 cup of brown rice, 1/2 cup snap beans
Herbal tea

8 raw oysters in lemon juice
1/2 cup potato salad
1 cup broccoli in apple cider vinegar and olive oil
Herbal tea

Drug Store and Health Food Aphrodisiacs For Men

Good multi-vitamin/mineral tablet or capsule
    once or twice daily
Lecithin capsules, two with meals
Fish oil capsules, one or two with meals
Garlic capsules, one or two with meals
Bee pollen, sprinkled on breakfast
Royal jelly tablets or capsules once or twice a day
Ginseng one or more times a day
Gotu Kola once a day

Drug Store and Health Food Aphrodisiacs For Women

Good multi-vitamin/mineral tablet or capsule
    once or twice daily
Lecithin capsules, two with meals
Fish oil capsules, one or two with meals
Garlic capsules, one or two with meals
Bee pollen sprinkled on breakfast
Royal jelly once a day
Dong Quai once or twice a day

Vitamins
That
Block Cancer

by Dr. William H. Lee

Vitamins That Block Cancer

Stop and think for a moment.

Suppose there are certain inexpensive substances you can buy without a doctor's prescription which can provide a shield against cancer?

Suppose there are hundreds of scientific tests, double-blind studies, proving the worth of those substances?

Suppose you know nothing about those substances?

What a frightening situation. Why could it exist in this enlightened era of scientific and medical investigation? Why could millions of dollars be spent on cancer research and, yet, substances which could prevent cancer be hidden from the public?

The truth is that there is a large body of research. The truth is that this research does demonstrate impressive cancer protection by a number of "natural" substances. The truth is that this research has been published in responsible medical journals such as the *New England Journal of Medicine, The Lancet, American Journal of Clinical Nutrition,* and others.

So why haven't you heard about those substances?

This chapter presents information collected from many authentic and highly regarded scientific publications. Every reasonable effort has been made to provide reliable scientific results and information. The sources of the research are documented so you may check the articles cited, but the author and publisher cannot assume responsibility for the consequence of their use. Readers are advised to consult a physician regarding any dietary modification.

Cancer Prevention
What is Cancer?

It has been described for thousands of years but, until recently, has been a mystery disease. For centuries, patients have been described who developed growths. For centuries it was known that those patients would weaken and die but it was not known why.

As better examination techniques came about (the microscope, etc.), the growths were found to be different from normal tissue. They were bizarrely formed with only a slight resemblance to the surrounding tissue. But what made them appear?

Cancer cells look different from normal cells. They also behave differently. Cancer cells divide like normal cells, but unlike normal cells they continue to divide without any restrictions and can invade distant areas and organs in the body. When normal cells are grown outside the body in a laboratory, they have a limited lifespan. They will divide a number of times and then die even though there is space and nutrient material for them to live on. This is considered normal and the cells are "mortal". However, cancer cells will continue to grow and divide in the laboratory for an indefinite period of time providing there is space to grow and nutrients to feed on. In that sense, cancer cells are "immortal".

Therefore, in the body, cancer cells need all of the space they can find. They expand into whatever tissue is around them and destroy it. The cells continue to divide. This growth requires nutrients and blood which the body supplies . . . and the body pays for its own continuing destruction.

Lack of Inhibition

Normal cells understand the laws of the body. When normal cells grow, they grow in a typical pattern and when they come in contact with another cell, they cease their growth. The law is called *contact inhibition*.

Cancer cells do not obey the law. When they make contact with another cell they continue to grow. They'll make masses of cells, clump one on another into ugly lumps and
mountains. They'll burrow into surrounding tissue like plants invading the soil. They'll push aside surrounding tissue to get at the nutrients they want.

How Do Normal Cells Become Cancer Cells?

It is now thought that all normal cells have the potential to become cancerous. All normal cells have genes called *oncogenes*, but they do not exert their influence until activated by cancer-causing-agents. Agents which activate cancer genes are called tumor promotors.

NOTE: Human beings are seldom exposed to high doses of tumor promotors or tumor initiators, but they are frequently exposed to low doses of these cancer causing substances.

DNA molecules are present in all cells. DNA molecules are called genes. Segments of genes responsible for cancer are called oncogenes.

Tumor initiators are chemicals which activate cancer-causing genes.

Tumor promoters are chemicals which further stimulate *already activated* cancer genes.

Laboratory experiments have shown that the combined influence of two initiators is more effective in producing cancer than the individual agents.

What Are These Initiators and Promoters of Cancer?

Ultraviolet light . . . radiation . . . asbestos . . . tobacco smoke . . . alcohol . . . excess fat . . . steroids . . . aflatoxins . . . chemotherapeutic agents . . . herbicides . . . pesticides . . . arsenic . . . cadmium . . . mercury . . . lead . . . nitrosamines . . . etc.

Frightening and Hopeful

It's frightening to know that all of our cells carry the seed of our own destruction.

It's hopeful because once you discover the cause you can more easily defeat it!

First, a look at how cancer patients are treated today:
1) toxic chemicals, 2) surgery, 3) radiation.

The "cure" is potentially at least as harmful as the disease.

Cancer Shields

Logic tells us that we can protect ourselves against cancer by eliminating those factors which stimulate the oncogenes.

Logic also tells us that, while we can eliminate those factors under our control (cigarettes, alcohol, excess fats, etc.), elimination of most of the rest of the factors from the environment and the diet requires legislation and extreme government intervention.

Therefore, while we will exert influence over what we can, we can also use other weapons that are available to us. They include dietary anticancer agents such as vitamins, minerals, trace minerals, protease inhibitors, fiber, and accessory nutrients.

We can now erect cancer shields by being careful of what we eat and by taking supplemental nutrients.

Many experiments have shown that there are several specific nutrients which reduce the risk of cancer from radiation and from chemical carcinogens. These anticancer nutrients include:

Vitamins

Vitamins A, C, E, Beta-carotene, B-Complex

Minerals

Selenium, Zinc

Amino Acids

L-Cysteine, methionine

Plus many more natural nutrients which will be revealed in the following pages detailing some of the studies done in leading universities.

NOTE: One marvelous book entitled, *Until A Cure Comes*, by Jay M. Davis, M.D., Ph.D., Miller Press, Eureka, CA., details the author's daily supplemental regimen. This is what he takes as a preventative routine along with diet modification:

Selenium 300 micrograms (slightly higher than the recommended daily allowance of 50 to 200 micrograms)

Vitamin E	400 I.U.
Beta-carotene	15 - 30 milligrams
Vitamin A	10,000 I.U.
Vitamin C	500 milligrams

Other dietary factors which serve to protect us include:
Lactobacillus acidophilus
Garlic and onions
Phytosterols
Omega 3 fatty acids
Omega 6 fatty acids
Calcium
Gamma linolenic acid, etc.

How Do Vitamins Help?

Vitamins A, E, C and Beta-carotene are potent anticancer agents which may reduce cancer risk in multiple ways, some of which are described.

Antioxidant Power

These vitamins have what we call "antioxidant" power: This means that they can shut down free radicals (extremely active molecules which cause cell death or the production of inadequate cells). Many cancer-causing agents generate these free radicals. But these vitamins, when in higher-than-normal amounts in the body, can combine with the free radicals and squelch their harmful activities.

Reduce The Formation and Amount of
Cancer-Causing Agents

Vitamins C and E may prevent the formation and/or reduce the level of cancer-causing agents in the stomach and intestines. For example: nitrites that are commonly used as a preservative in various foods such as hot dogs, sausage, cured meats, salads, etc. Nitrites are not cancer-causing by themselves but when combined with amines naturally present in the body, they form potent cancer-causing agents called nitrosamines.

The equation looks like this:

Nitrites + Amines = Nitrosamines

Nitrosamines are water soluble and since the body operates on waterways (the bloodstream) the cancerous agents can be carried anywhere.

When vitamin C and/or vitamin E is present in copious amounts the equation changes to:

Nitrites + Amines + vitamin C or E = little or no Nitrosamine

Therefore, if you want to eat a hot dog and just can't do without it, protect yourself by taking some vitamin C or vitamin E to reduce its production of cancer-causing nitrosamines. How much will you need as a preventive agent? Nobody knows exactly how much vitamin C or E is needed but 200 milligrams of C and about 50 I.U. of vitamin E should be adequate for a hot dog with mustard and sauerkraut.

Nitrosamines are just one of many mutagenic substances (substances which influence genetic changes that may or may not lead to cancer) which are formed in the stomach and the rest of the intestinal tract. Changes in genetic material precede cancer formation. The level of mutagenic substances found in the waste material of meat eaters is higher than that found in the waste material of vegetarians. Seventh Day Adventists, who are vegetarians, have a much lower incidence of cancer than meat-eating groups. Taking supplements of vitamin C or vitamin E reduces the levels of mutagens discovered in the waste material of meat eaters.

Furthermore, taking both vitamin C and E is more effective than taking either of them individually. Some nutritionists think that taking vitamin C 500 milligrams a day and vitamin E 400 I.U. a day can be effective against developing polyps, a precursor of colon cancer. More tests will be needed to discover the individual needs for these vitamins since some people may respond better to a higher dose of vitamin C along with the vitamin E.

Most malignant chemicals cannot cause cancer unless they are converted to an active form. The following vitamins can prevent that conversion from inactive to active form: Vitamins A, C, E, and Beta-carotene.

Can We Get Enough Of These Vitamins From Food?

Medical authorities say yes.

Many nutritionists say no!

In order to inhibit the change from inactive form to active form you must have high levels of the vitamins present in the body at the same time that the chemicals are present. We eat three times a day at least. We drink water a number of times a day, we breathe in pollutants 24 hours a day. Because vitamins A and E are oil-soluble vitamins, they can be stored in the body, but vitamin C is water-soluble and is lost very quickly. So, not only do you have to replenish it daily, but possibly a number of times a day.

In order to obtain all of the vitamins you need to do their regular jobs in the body and to protect against cancer, you'd have to do nothing but eat the best of foods all day long. I think that supplements are the answer.

How Else Do Vitamins Help?

Some experiments suggest that the cancer-fighters can convert newly formed cancer cells back to normal cells.

Vitamin C has been shown to change new chemically-induced cancer cells back to normal cells.

Vitamin A has been shown to transform some well established cancer cells to cells resembling normal cells.

Vitamin E has also transformed established skin cancer cells to normal cells.

While the exact amounts of vitamins needed to reverse cancer cells to normal cells varies from individual to individual, the doses of vitamin A, E, and C shown in this chapter are known to be helpful.

Vitamins Stimulate Your Body's
Immune Defense Against Cancer

Large amounts of vitamins A, E, C, Beta-carotene and other nutrients have been shown to stimulate the body's defense system — which in turn will kill newly-formed cancer cells. If these new-formed cells are killed before they can grow and spread, a cancer-free state may be established.

Some studies have shown that vitamin C (up to 4 grams daily), vitamin E (up to 1200 I.U. daily), vitamin A (up to 12000 I.U. daily), and Beta-carotene (up to 10,000 units daily) stimulate the body's defense system.

Many of the above doses are based on animal studies and have been criticized because the doses of carcinogens which produce tumors in animals are generally higher than those which humans are exposed to. However, although humans are not exposed to high doses of single carcinogens daily, they are exposed to multiple carcinogens in low doses every day of their lives. And, if you remember, multiple exposure is more likely to trigger the oncogenes than single exposures.

Critics abound and if mankind is going to wait around until proof positive satisfies everybody, there will be a lot less of us to enjoy the proof. In addition, the rest of this chapter will illustrate some of the human studies that have convinced many experts that real cancer cure depends on prevention.

In my opinion, you have to take supplements. Vitamins A, C, E, Beta-carotene, L-cysteine and L-methionine are target nutrients. Their job is to protect you against disease and to reinforce immune protection inside your body. Many other nutrients have also demonstrated the ability to support this fight. Among them are the B-vitamins, zinc, calcium and magnesium. And, one of the most important is the mineral selenium.

There are more than 50 nutrients found in food which are needed daily to energize, repair, rejuvenate and protect your body. Some of the nutrients can be obtained from the foods you eat but others are more difficult to obtain. Selenium supplementation is a must. Because of its free radical scavenging, and its contributions to cell oxygen uptake, and its neutralization of toxins and carcinogens, selenium is in the forefront of cancer fighters.

Vitamin C is not only an antioxidant but stimulates the immune system, decreases blood cholesterol levels, fights stress and cancer cells.

L-cysteine is a sulfur-bearing amino acid which is a potent antioxidant and is essential for oxygen transport. It should be taken with 2 to 3 times its amount of vitamin C. (L-cysteine 500 milligrams with vitamin C 1500 milligrams daily.) The other protective amino acid, L-methionine, is also, along with L-cysteine, a precursor of glutathione peroxidase. Glutathione peroxidase is one member of the body's main natural defense team.

All of these nutrients can be found in antioxidant formulas available at health or drugstores. Use them with a diet which includes foods having a natural content of cancer fighters. These foods include:

Vitamin A

Cantaloupe, apricots, mangoes, liver, eggs, milk

Beta-carotene

Yellow vegetables and fruit, cabbage, lettuce, spinach

Vitamin C

Oranges, lemons, limes, pineapples, raspberries, strawberries, grapefruit, brussel sprouts, cauliflower, peas, cabbage, green peppers

Vitamin E

Fish, apples, tomatoes, cucumbers, almonds, spinach, parsley, mustard greens, turnip greens, sweet potatoes

(This is just a small listing of helpful foods since many books have been written about foods and their nutrient content.)

1. Eat a variety of foods.
2. Reduce your consumption of sugar and salt.
3. Avoid too much fat, saturated fat and cholesterol.
4. Make unprocessed carbohydrates, fresh fruits and vegetables, whole grains and legumes, the major part of your diet.
5. Decrease meat consumption and increase fish eating and poultry.
6. Don't overeat.

Quotes From Journals

"Folic Acid and Cervical Cancer" *Acta Cytologica* 1987:31:697

Symptoms of folic acid deficiency often accompany cervical cancer or precancerous states, report researchers at Emory University in Atlanta.

Results show folic acid deficiency (one of the B-Complex vitamins) is accompanied by concomitant cancer-like changes in cervical tissue.

"Lactobacteria Bulgaricus Capable of Inhibiting Tumors" *JNCI* 77:633, 1986

Several Russian investigators have isolated antitumor nutrient compounds from the cell wall of L. bulgaricus capable of inhibiting proliferation of tumors in laboratory animals. A control study of nearly 3,000 subjects that analyzed consumption of alcohol and dairy products found that eating yogurt was associated with a dramatic drop in the incidence of breast cancer.

"Vitamin C Treatment/Aids" *Med. Hypotheses* 14:423-433, Aug. 1984

The amount of vitamin C that can be tolerated without producing diarrhea is markedly increased by viral illnesses. Preliminary evidence from patients with acquired immune deficiency syndrome

(AIDS) suggests that treatment with vitamin C, titrated to bowel tolerance, can produce remission of symptoms and decreased tendency to secondary infection, although helper/suppressor T-cells ratios remain depressed. A topical vitamin C paste or solution has been effective for AIDS-related herpes simplex.

"Cancer and Vitamin A" *Cancer Res.* 46:5264-5269, Oct. 1986
Rats were given vitamin A for two weeks before being exposed to a carcinogen and were supplemented for an additional six months after exposure. The supplemented rats had 37% fewer cancers.

"Lung Cancer, Vitamin A/Carotene" *American Journal of Epidemiolology* 120: 769-776, Nov. 1984
A pattern seems to be emerging from this study and other studies of a protective effect of vitamin A and/or Beta-carotene in sites where squamous cell histological types of lung cancer prevail.

"Cervical Cancer/Carotene Intake" *International Journal of Cancer* 34:319-322, Sept. 1984
Consumption of carrots and of green vegetables, as well as Beta-carotene, lowered the risk of cervical cancer. Beta-carotene or some other aspect of a vegetable-rich diet appears to be protective against invasive cervical cancer.

"Vitamin A/Radiation Injury" *Ann.Surg.* 200:494-512, Oct. 1984
A non-toxic amount of vitamin A was added to the diet of rats within two days of a damaging dose of whole-body gamma radiation. The incidence of radiation-induced ulcers was reduced by as much as 78%. Previous experiments have shown that vitamin A, as well as Beta-carotene, increases antitumor action.

"The Bacteria in Yogurt May Help Prevent Colon Cancer" *American Journal of Clinical Nutrition* 39:756-61, 1984
21 healthy human subjects were fed viable lactobacillus acidophilus and the feces were analyzed for concentrations of bacterial

enzymes known to change precancerous cells to cancer cells. Those enzymes were significantly reduced after only one month of supplementation.

"Garlic or Onion May Inhibit Tumor Growth" *Carcinogenesis* 4(8):1063-5, 1983
Garlic oil and onion oil were equally effective in decreasing the number and incidence of skin tumors.

"Omega 3 Fatty Acids" *Nutrition and Cancer* 6:254-9, 1984
Dietary fish oil may inhibit the development of breast cancer.

"Omega 6 Fatty Acids" *Medical Hypothesis* 6:469-86, 1980
May actually reverse cancer growth by restoring prostaglandin E series metabolism.

Am. J. Obstet. & Gyn. 151:632-5, 1985
Observational study revealed that plasma Beta-carotene level was significantly lower in cervical cancer patients.

Int. J. Cancer vol. 34:319-22, 1984
Observational study suggests that either dietary Beta-carotene or some related aspect of a vegetable-rich diet is protective against cervical cancer.

Lancet, Nov. 28, 1981, pp. 1185-90
In a 19 year study of almost 2,000 men, the intake of Beta-carotene was inversely related to the incidence of lung cancer.

J. Nat. Cancer Inst. 73:1463-8, 1984
In a survey of over 6,000 people, low Beta-carotene levels were correlated with lung cancer mortality.

JAMA 226:1421-1424, 1973
In clinical test after clinical test, cervical cells of women using oral contraceptive agents showed pre-cancerous features. But these

pre-cancerous cells disappeared when these women were given oral folate supplementation.

Am. J. Clin. Nutr. 35:73-82, 1982

47 women on birth control pills who had a pre-cancerous condition received either 10 milligrams oral folic acid daily or a placebo. After three months, cervical biopsies *showed a significant improvement only in the women receiving the vitamin.* 4 women on the placebo (a pill that looks like folic acid but contains none of the vitamin) developed cancer.

Med. Hypotheses 16:421-8, 1985

Theoretical discussion. Since vitamin B-6 is a co-enzyme in the biosynthesis of thymidine, a deficiency of which can increase mutagenesis, a B-6 deficiency along with contact with carcinogens could lead to tumor initiation.

Am. J. Epidemiol. 113(6):675-80, 1981

In a study of 374 males with cancer of the larynx and 381 controls, those ingesting low amounts of vitamin A in their diets had twice the risk of those ingesting large amounts of vitamin A.

Brit. J. Urology, 55(5):525-8, 1983

In 19 patients with prostate cancer, serum zinc was significantly lower than in 27 patients with prostatic hyperplasia and there was a significant zinc/vitamin A correlation.

J. Nat. Cancer Inst. 73:1463-6, 1984

Observational Study. In a survey of over 6,000 people, low vitamin A levels were associated with death from stomach cancer.

Nutrition and Cancer 6(1):49-57, 1984

Women consuming less than average vitamin A and Beta-carotene were three times as likely to develop severe dysplasia and 2-3/4 times as likely to develop carcinoma.

J. Nat. Cancer Instit. 73:1463-8, 1984
Observational study. In a survey of 6,000 people, vitamin C levels were lower in all cancer groups and especially lower in those dying from gastric cancer.

Proc. Nat. Acad. Sci. USA 75:4538-42, 1978
Vitamin C 10 grams daily in divided doses were given orally to "hopelessly ill" patients. Mean survival times were 300 days longer when compared to historical controls. Survival for more than one year after the date of "untreatability" was observed in 22% of the experimental group but in only .4% of the control group.

Life Sci. 21(2):275-80, 1980
Vitamin C may block the formation of carcinogenic nitrosamines to protect against stomach cancer.

Carcinogenisis 6(11):1675-76, 1985
8 volunteers received ascorbic acid (vitamin C) 1 gram daily. Levels of mutagenic substances in the gastric juice were significantly lower after one week, suggesting that vitamin C supplementation may significantly reduce the levels of genotoxic chemicals in gastric juice.

Cancer Res. 45:6519-22, 1985
Vitamin C. 2 grams daily was effective in blocking the formation of nitrosamines in 10 students fed nitrate and proline.

Exp. Cell Biology, 47(3):210-17, 1979
Vitamin B-12 and vitamin C may inhibit carcinogens when given together.

Brit. J. Cancer 49:321-4 1984
Observational Study. In a study of 5004 women, those who developed breast cancer had a mean plasma vitamin E level that was significantly lower than controls.

Am. J. Clin. Nutr. 33:2511-12, 1980
Vitamin E supplements reduced the cancer-causing agents found in the stool by as much as 79%.

Science News, 3/2/85 p. 141
People drinking soft water (low in calcium) have more colon cancer, while those eating high calcium diets have less colon cancer.

Lancet 1:307-9, 1985
Observational Study. In a study of 1,954 men, those with the lowest combined index of calcium and vitamin D were 2-1/2 times more likely to develop colorectal cancer.

Carcinogenesis 1:199, 1980
Selenium prevented or delayed the appearance of breast tumors in mice infected with a carcinogenic virus.

Brit. J. Urology 55(5):525:8, 1983
Observational Study. 19 patients with prostatic carcinoma had significantly lower levels of zinc in the serum than 27 patients with benign prostatic hypertrophy.

Am. J. Clin. Nutr. 40(4 suppl.):927-30, 1984
Phytosterols (cholesterol analogs found in plants) may be protective against colon cancer.

Cancer Res. 45:3311-21, July, 1985
Vitamin A could be used to prevent cancer spread by keeping tumor cells trapped in their original area.

Rowett Research Institute, Scotland (Your Health, Jan. 3, 1989)
Vitamin E shows potential in warding off cell deterioration. A daily dose of 1000 I.U. helps guard smokers against lung cancer by preventing damage caused by "free radicals" which can harm cells and cause lung cancer.

A study comparing smokers and non-smokers found that the smokers red blood cells were three times more susceptible to cell damage than non-smokers. *However, smokers on vitamin E were as resistant as non-smokers.*

U.S. Agriculture Department Human Nutrition Research Center on Aging
A study showed *800 milligrams of vitamin E daily* seems to *bolster immune systems* which lose disease-fighting ability with age. *It may therefore help elderly people fend off infections and other diseases.*

J. Nutr. Growth Cancer 1:207-10, July-Dec. 1984
Vitamin B-1 supplementation could help prevent cell damage, fibrinogenesis, and collagen breakdown in cancer patients.

J. Nutr. 114:938-945, May, 1984
Vitamin B-6 deficiency increases susceptibility to onogenesis by impairing the immune response.

JNCI 73:767-770, Sept. 1984
Niacinamide (vitamin B-3) inhibited cancer development simultaneously at several places in the body and is effective against more than one class of carcinogen. It may act by stimulating the repair of damaged DNA.

Nutr. Cancer 6:13-21, Mar. 1984
Selenium/skin cancer. Although the mechanism is not known, the hypothesis is that higher selenium levels reduce the risk of developing some cancers.

J. Agricultural Food Chem. 32:436-442, May-June 1984
Anti-cancer properties of selenium are reviewed. Selenium should be considered not only as a preventive, but also as a curative agent in cancer treatment and may act additively or synergistically with drug and x-ray treatments (this also might be said in regard to prostate cancer).

JNCI 72:419-425, Feb. 1984

Dietary zinc deficiency, in conjunction with high levels of nitrosamines or their precursors, may be a factor in the etiology of human esophageal cancer.

Med. 15:15-33, Jul. 1984

The effect of fatty acids on the growth of cultured human osteogenic sarcoma cells was examined. Linolenic acid, linoleic acid, eicosapentaenoic acid and docosahexaenoic acid all had growth suppressive effects. (Those fatty acids are found in vegetable oil and in fish oil.)

Arachidonic acid and GLA also showed suppressive activity. Prostaglandin activity may be involved in the inhibitory effects of polyunsaturated fatty acids on cancer growth.

JNCI 74:1145-1150, May, 1985

Fatty acid analysis of tumor and hepatic microsomal lipids showed that fish oil levels were inversely related to mammary tumor development. In other words, the more fatty acids, the fewer breast tumors.

Am. J. Chinese Med. 11:69-73, 1983

Mice were fed diets supplemented with garlic for 4 days before being inoculated with tumor cells. The proliferation of tumor cells, measured after ten days was decreased by 20 to as much as 51% in mice fed ground fresh garlic.

Vitamin C, Selenium, and Hypertension

The authors studied the relationship between plasma vitamin C levels, serum selenium, and hypertension in 722 Finnish men. Higher serum vitamin C levels were associated with lower blood pressure, both systolic and diastolic. A higher serum selenium level was also associated with lower blood pressure.

"The marked elevation of blood pressure at the lowest levels of plasma ascorbic acid and serum selenium concentrations supports the hypothesis that antioxidants play a role in the etiology of hypertension."

Jukka T. Salonen, Riitta Salonen, Merja Ihanainen, Markku Parviainen, Ritva Seppanen, Marjatta Kantola, Kari Seppanen, Rainer Rauramaa. "Blood pressure, dietary fats, and antioxidants." *American Journal of Clinical Nutrition* 48:1226-1232 (November 1988). University of Kuopio, P.O. Box 6, 70211 Kuopio, Finland (J.T. Salonon).

Carotene and Cancer

Cancer of the larynx is a squamous cell cancer, comparable to squamous cell lung cancer. Since carotene and vitamin A appear to have a protective effect against squamous cell lung cancer, the authors studied the relationship of carotene and vitamin A intake to cancer of the larynx.

Dietary interviews were conducted with 151 men with cancer of the larynx and 178 controls, in six counties in Texas. The interview was based on a food frequency questionnaire containing 42 foods or types of foods which are major contributors to vitamin A intake.

A low total vitamin A intake or a low retinol intake was not related to cancer risk. However, a low carotene intake increased the odds ratio for cancer by two-fold. (Thus, a high carotene intake appeared to be protective against cancer of the larynx.)

There was an 11-fold increase in risk for cancer of the larynx in smokers. A high carotene intake was protective in men who had stopped smoking, but not in smokers.

"Although increased carotene intake could be encouraged as part of a smoking cessation program, the public should not be given the impression that increasing carotene consumption is an effective way to reduce the risk of respiratory cancer in the presence of continued smoking."

Dorothy Mackerras, Patricia A. Buffler, D. Elizabeth Randall, Milton Z. Nichaman, Linda W. Pickle, Thomas J. Mason. "Carotene intake and the risk of laryngeal cancer in coastal Texas." *American Journal of Epidemiology* 128:980-988 (1988). School of Public Health, University of Texas Health Science Center, Houston, Texas 77225 (P.A. Buffler).

Vitamins A and C
and Lung Cancer

The authors report the results of a case-control study of 1253 lung cancer patients and 1274 controls in southern Louisiana. A higher carotene intake was associated with a lower cancer risk, as has been reported in previous studies. Somewhat surprisingly, a stronger protective effect was associated with vitamin C intake. The protective effects were limited to squamous cell and small cell lung cancer.

Elizabeth T. H. Fonthan, Linda Williams Pickle, William Haenszel, Pelayo Correa, Youping Lin, Roni T. Falk. "Dietary vitamins A and C and lung cancer risk in Louisiana." *Cancer* 62: 2267-2273 (November 15, 1988). Department of Pathology, Louisiana State University Medical Center, 1901 Perdido Street, New Orleans, Louisiana 70112 (E.T.H. Foatham).

Vitamin E And Cancer

"Vitamin E may protect against cancer by functioning as an intracellular antioxidant and as a free radical scavenger." Animal studies and human epidemiological studies are contradictory, perhaps because vitamin E may be protective only against certain types of cancers.

The author studied the relationship between serum vitamin E levels and various types of cancers among women in Finland. Data were collected on 313 cancer cases and 578 controls, from a massive screening program conducted in 1966-1972.

"Women with low serum alpha-tocopherol levels had a higher risk of cancer than other women, especially in the sub-category of epithelial cancers." The author suggests that "a low vitamin E intake is a risk factor for cancer in many, but not all, organs."

Paul Knekt. "Serum vitamin E level and risk of female cancers." *International Journal of Epidemiology* 17:281-286 (1988). Research Institute for Social Security, P.O. Box 78, SF-00381, Helsinki, Finland.

Serum Levels of Beta-carotene

There is substantial evidence suggesting that beta-carotene has a protective effect against cancer. The University of Pittsburgh is undertaking trial of the cancer-protecting effect of beta-carotene in men at high risk for lung cancer. Over 400 men have been recruited, all of them smokers of at least a pack a day for at least 20 years.

This report concerns serum beta-carotene levels in 150 men who were given 15 mg of beta-carotene per day for 10 months. "After 4 months of treatment, the average serum beta-carotene level increased 10-fold and the average carotenoid level more than doubled." There was no further significant increase in the remaining 6 months of treatment. None of the men reported yellowing of the skin or any other side effects.

"These findings indicate that if effective against cancer beta-carotene would be an ideal chemopreventive agent. It is relatively inexpensive, easy to administer, and at least under the conditions of this study has no side effects."

Joseph P. Costantino, Lewis H. Kuller, Lisa Begg, Carol K. Redmond, Margaret W. Bates. "Serum level changes after administration of a pharmacologic dose of beta-carotene." *American Journal of Clinical Nutrition* 48:1277-1283 (November 1988). Room 326 Parran Hall, Graduate School of Public Health, University of Pittsburgh, Pittsburgh, Pennsylvania 15261 (J.P. Costantino).

Why Take Supplements
& How Much?

We can't manufacture our own vitamins. We can't make vitamins A, C, and E . . . we must get them from external sources. The vitamin A, whether from food or supplements, is only about 10% to 20% used by the body because our efficiency is not that good.

The highest vitamin A activity is about 3 to 6 hours after ingestion. In about 12 hours, the level drops off so, in spite of the fact that it is stored in the body, it's a good idea to take vitamin A once a day and Beta-carotene (the precursor of vitamin A — the body changes it into usable vitamin A if needed) once a day. Take one in the morning and the other 12 hours later.

When we take vitamin C, only a certain percentage will be usable. A 500 milligram dose will be about 50% usable. The vitamin C is rapidly dispersed throughout the body and rapidly lost through waste. Either take it four times a day or take a good time-dispersed vitamin C formula that will stay in the body for ten to twelve hours.

Vitamin E is about 20% bioavailable, peaks in about 4 to 6 hours and hits its lowest level in about 12 hours. Perhaps the best way to insure protection is to take it in divided doses twice a day.

Dr. Linus Pauling in his book, "How To Live Longer and Feel Better," Freeman and Co., N.Y., 1986, takes on the task of developing the quantities of supplements needed for your basic defense system. Since all vitamins work together, he's listed a basic vitamin formula on the following page which compares the recommendations of 4 nutritional experts with the RDA (recommended daily allowance).

You will have to choose your quantities depending on which expert is most appealing to you.

Although not mentioned, selenium, Beta-carotene and zinc supplements are in the following neighborhood:

Selenium	50 to 200 micrograms daily
Beta-carotene	10000 I.U. daily
Zinc	25 milligrams daily

A good multi-vitamin/mineral will have a number of these nutrients in the indicated amounts. A good antioxidant formula will usually supply appropriate amounts of vitamin A, C, E plus selenium, zinc and Beta-carotene.

Vitamin Fixes
To Go Along With Supplements

You want to obtain vitamins naturally as well as from supplements so your body retains the ability to extract vitamins from foods and utilize them naturally. Here are a few vitamin fixes to start you on the way.

Vitamin A Fix

1 cup cantaloupe
1 raw carrot
1 cup broccoli
1 cup turnip greens
about 35,000 I.U. of vitamin A in total

Vitamin C Fix

1 orange
1 cup strawberries
1/2 cup papaya
1 cup canned tomato soup
1 kiwi
about 400 milligrams of vitamin C in total

	RDA	WILLIAMS	ALLEN	LEIBOVITZ	PAULING
Vitamin C	60 mg	2500 mg	1500 mg	2500 mg	1000-18000 mg
Vitamin E	10 IU	400 IU	600 IU	300 IU	800 IU
Vitamin A	5000 IU	15000 IU	15000IU	20000 IU	20-40000 IU
Vitamin K	None	100 mg	None	None	None
Vitamin D	400 IU	400 IU	300 IU	800 IU	800 IU
B-1	1.5 mg	20 mg	300 mg	100 mg	50-100 mg
B-2	1.7 mg	20 mg	200 mg	100 mg	50-100 mg
B-3	18 mg	200 mg	750 mg	300 mg	300-600 mg
B-6	2.2 mg	30 mg	350 mg	100 mg	50-100 mg
B-12	3 mg	90 mg	1000 mg	100 mg	100-200 mg
Folacin	400 mg	400 mg	400 mg	400 mg	400-800 mg
Pantothenic Acid	None	150 mg	500 mg	200 mg	100-200 mg

Calcium Fix

3 oz. canned sardines
1 cup yogurt
1 cup skim milk
1 cup cooked spinach
1 oz. cheddar cheese
about 1500 milligrams of calcium in total

B-Vitamin Fix

Any combination which adds up to 4 to 6 servings of B-rich foods:

3/4 cup bran
1 slice of whole grain bread
1/2 cup brown rice
1/2 cup peas
3 oz. tuna
1/2 cup lentils
1 oz. almonds
3 oz. turkey
1/2 cup cottage cheese

Protein Fix

Proteins are needed because they are the raw materials from which the immune system fighters are made.

6 to 8 oz. of protein foods daily
salmon, sole, trout, tuna
skinless poultry
lean meat
eggs, beans, rice
tofu

Questions & Answers

When is the best time to take vitamins?

With meals. Vitamins are concentrated foods and the body has to handle the digestion and assimilation the same way it absorbs food. If you take your vitamin/mineral supplements in the morning with just a cup of coffee, you might as well not bother to take a supplement at all.

When it comes to supplements, is more better?

Not so. You can take too much of a good thing. Vitamin A, in excess of 100,000 I.U. daily for any length of time can possibly do some damage to the body. An excess of zinc can deplete the body of copper. As with any therapy, good sense is important.

Does my doctor know all there is to know about vitamins?

Not usually, unless he or she is an exceptional person who has taken the time to study *after medical school.* Most medical schools do not teach the use of vitamins for treatment or for the prevention of disease.

Where can I get information about vitamin therapy?

For the most part you'll have to do a lot of reading for yourself and search out a nutritionally-oriented physician. Some health food stores are helpful and so are some pharmacists.

Do I have to take supplements all of the time or just when I have a cold or feel sick?

When is the best time to dig a well? Before or after you feel thirsty? When is the best time to make a plow? Figure it out for yourself . . .

I know that vegetarians may be healthier than meat eaters but I like to eat meat.

While it is true that eating meat has been linked to colon cancer, meat is also an important source of nutrients. Therefore, the answer is moderation. Eat some meat but substitute fish and chicken for some of the meat meals. In that way you'll cut the cancer risk and still be able to enjoy a meat dish.

My doctors say a "balanced diet" is all I need and that supplements are a bunch of bunk.

A balanced diet may provide you with enough nutrients to carry on work and/or play (if there is such a thing as a "balanced diet") but probably not enough nutrients to protect you against cancer. This is because the "balanced" diet simply does not have enough power to fight the constantly emerging stream of free radicals. Also, why is it that doctors die about 15% earlier than other people?

Is it true that a lot of the vitamins I take are lost in the urine?

Probably so. If you take more than the body needs at the time, particularly the water soluble vitamin C and the B-Complex, you will lose some in the urine. But remember that they are bathing the various body parts as they are leaving and may be a protection even then!

The Wonders
of Internal
Cleansing

Wash Invisible Poisons
Right Out Of Your Body

Dr. William H. Lee

It's a Jungle Out There . . .
And in Here as Well!

We have ancient bodies in a space-age world.

In the last 10,000 to 25,000 years, the human body has changed very little but we are exposed to literally thousands of chemical compounds — many of them toxic — that our ancestors never contacted in their lives.

The body's built-in mechanisms to handle toxic substances have become outdated!

For the most part, the toxic substances our ancestors had to worry about were edible. If they ate or drank a substance that was harmful, the body was designed to protect itself. The body's first line of defense has always been the sense of taste. We tend to reject foods that do not "taste right". The second line of defense, the stomach. Toxins are gotten rid of through vomiting or diarrhea. And the third line of defense has always been the liver. It filters toxins out of the bloodstream, renders them harmless and puts them in storage or excretes them through the kidneys.

Because of these built-in systems, most of the toxins the body has become familiar with over the centuries are easily managed. Spoiled foods are usually rejected by the stomach or the taste buds. A small amount of alcohol can be neutralized by special enzymes produced by the liver cells and changed into substances the body can use or excrete.

However, our natural defenses need help now.

They are not so effective against modern toxins. Our physical systems simply have not had the time necessary to adapt to the multitude of chemical pesticides, preservatives, flavors, colors, radiation, smog, smoke, automobile exhaust, and other pollutants we are exposed to nowadays.

The millenia it takes for the human body to adapt to changes will certainly not help those of us living now. It is up to us to learn how to manipulate our diet to cleanse the body tissues of the effects of deadly toxins with vitamin and mineral substances which are helpful.

In the last 100 years, although we have been able to control the infectious diseases such as small pox, typhoid fever, diphtheria, etc., many other diseases have increased.

Myocardial Infarction (heart attack). More than a million deaths a year.

Diabetes Mellitus. Incidence has increased with nine million diabetics in the U.S.

Osteoporosis. Thirty percent of women over 50 are at increased risk of hip fracture from bone loss. In less developed areas of the world this condition is practically unheard of.

Hyperactivity. This disorder was unheard of twenty years ago. Now it is found in more than one-half million children.

Kidney stones. In the U.S., the incidence has doubled in the past twenty years.

Diverticulosis, diverticulitis, colon cancer. Practicing in Africa for thirty years, Dennis Burkitt, M.D. did not see these conditions which are epidemic in the U.S.

Intestinal disorders. Belching, bloating, and irritable bowel syndrome. Very common. Two million have ulcerative colitis, which is unheard of in certain areas of the world.

Prostate problems. Seventy percent of older men have enlarged prostate glands which may require surgery.

Cholesterol, liver damage, free radical damage, damage from the sun . . .

There are three main ways toxins can enter our bodies and cause trouble. In the air we breathe, through our skin, and through our food and water.

We can't give up breathing, eating and drinking, and we need our skin to hold us together. So, we will have to learn to help our body's natural defense systems stay at maximum power and also learn how to effectively neutralize as many toxic substances as possible, or convert them into useful or inert substances.

Some of the answers are in this chapter . . . unfortunately, not all of the answers are to be found anywhere.

Do Your Part In Keeping Your Food
Safer To Eat

Our health and perhaps our lives are being threatened by the food we eat, say top researchers. The pesticides used to protect our food from insects and spoilage are attacking us. While fruits and vegetables have received the most press coverage, scientists are also reporting serious problems with beef, poultry, eggs, fish, shellfish and corn.

We are threatened almost daily with another new cancer-causing agent or other health hazard. According to the Natural Resources Defense Council (NRDC), between five thousand and six thousand American preschoolers may eventually get cancer, solely because of their exposure before the ages of six to eight to the pesticides commonly found in fruits and vegetables.

But there's more:

NRDC researchers estimate that at least three million pre-schoolers receive exposure to neurotoxic organophosphate insecticides from raw fruits and vegetables that are way above levels considered safe by the government.

In fact, the federal government found that fifty percent of all fruits have detectable levels of pesticides. Until there is some government action you have to learn to protect yourself!

Ways to Reduce Pesticide Risks

Two of the best ways to avoid pesticide residue, according to the Natural Resources Defense Council, is to buy domestically grown produce, and to buy produce in season. This ensures that the produce hasn't been stored for long periods, and thus is less likely to have been treated with pesticides, fungicides and other chemicals.

The chart on the following pages lists 15 of the most popular fruits and vegetables sold in the U.S., their growing seasons and how best to handle them.

PRODUCE	U.S. SEASON	PROPER HANDLING
APPLES	All Year	Wash with water. Keep cold and humid.
BANANAS	None	Avoid grayish-yellow fruit, which indicates chilling injury. Ripen at room temperature. Wash skin, peel and eat or refrigerate.
BROCCOLI	June-Nov.	Avoid those with yellow and wilted leaves, which indicate aging. Wash before using.
CARROTS	February-July	Buy firm, well-shaped roots with good orange color. Wash and brush before using.
CELERY	April-July, Oct.-Dec.	Choose thick, crisp, solid stalks. Wash before using.
GRAPEFRUIT	All year	Pick firm, not puffy or loose-skinned. Reddening or green tinge does not affect quality. Refrigerate or keep at room temperature. Wash.
GRAPES	June-January	Grapes won't increase in sweetness, so don't hold for further ripening. Rinse, refrigerate and use within one week.
LETTUCE	January-June	Select clean, firm heads that give slightly when squeezed. Twist to remove the core, rinse under running water. Drain. Store in tightly closed plastic bag or lettuce crisper.

PRODUCE	U.S. SEASON	PROPER HANDLING
ONIONS	May-November	Avoid those with soggy necks, soft or spongy bulbs indicating decay. Keep at room temperature in well ventilated, dry area. May be refrigerated. Store up to four weeks. Peel; wash before using.
ORANGES	All Year	Green skin color or reddening does not affect quality. Store at room temperature or refrigerate. Wash skin.
PEACHES	June-Sept.	Avoid green-tinged fruits and those that are hard, dull or bruised. Wash, hold at room temperature to soften, then refrigerate. Use promptly.
PEARS	Year-round, depending on variety.	Hold at room temperature for additional ripening, then refrigerate. Wash.
POTATOES	Year-round	Choose clean, smooth potatoes free of cuts or bruises. Avoid green-tinged potatoes. Never refrigerate; keep in cool, dry, well-ventilated dark area. Wash with brush and water.
SWEET CORN	May-November	Husk should be green, not dry or yellow. Shuck; wash before using.
TOMATOES	July-October	Place away from direct sunlight. Put in a paper bag to ripen. When ripe, wash; refrigerate; use within a few days.

Free Radicals

The headline in the *New York Times, Science Times* section, Tuesday, April 26, 1988, was startling: *Natural Chemicals Now Called Major Cause of Disease*, by Jane E. Brody.

Nutritionists had been warning about the problem of free radicals (highly reactive substances — produced both naturally and by industry) for years, but it was amazing to find it being told to the public in such graphic terms.

Free radical damage to the body is now explaining the damage done by tobacco smoke, sunlight, chemical carcinogens, fats in the blood and ozone in the air. Free oxygen radicals, the main type formed in living organisms, have been implicated in recent studies in more than sixty disorders including Alzheimers, Parkinson's, cataracts and rheumatoid arthritis. And, according to the leading authorities on aging, they contribute to many of the hallmarks of senescence such as wrinkling or lining of the skin, decline of kidney function and increased susceptibility to autoimmune diseases.

"The further along we get, the more overwhelmed we are by the number of disease states that involve free radicals," says Dr. Joel M. McCord, biochemist at the University of Southern Alabama College of Medicine. His discovery of a natural enzyme that helps disarm oxygen radicals allowed the first clear demonstration of the important role these substances play in the defense of the body.

Dr. McCord added that free radicals may not be the whole answer but may be important components in many different states and disorders.

Thus, in addition to causing disease directly, free radicals may set the stage for a disease caused by other factors. In other disease states they may make a disorder worse and in still others they may interfere with the body's natural healing process.

What are Free Radicals?

They are not the Chicago Seven!

They are electrically charged molecules in which the number of electrons, which have a negative charge, does not match the number of positively charged protons in the nucleus. They are therefore unstable and highly reactive because they must balance their electron configuration to match the positive charge.

Basically, what this means in simple language, is that a free radical is a madman — a rapist molecule — which will attack any body cell in order to steal an electron to satisfy its instability.

When it does that, it makes the cell, from which it stole an electron, a sick cell. If it happens to be a part of the nucleus which controls reproduction, then the sick cell will reproduce sick cells and, eventually, sicken the body. One free radical can set up a chain reaction that can damage critical molecules and ultimately kill cells. The body constantly attempts to prevent this damage with enzymes that block the formation of free radicals.

Among the important body chemicals which may be attacked by free radicals are vital enzymes, collagen (the cement that holds the body together), joints, neuro-transmitters in the brain, nucleic acids in the genetic material, perhaps causing mutations, and fatty acids which are the major components of cell membrane. When fat in the cell membrane is oxidized by free radicals to form lipid peroxides (the process by which fats become rancid), the integrity of the cell is destroyed rendering the cell as vulnerable to penetration as a house would be if the doors and windows were left open.

Lipid peroxides themselves are potent chemicals which can cause cellular damage, hinder metabolism, and reduce the flow of blood in tissues.

So, not only can free radicals cause trouble by themselves, but the by-products are also trouble-makers!

Where Do They Come From?

Oxygen is vital to our body. We can't live without it. However, too much or too little oxygen can create toxic by-products. The free radicals come from both internal and external sources. Internally, they are formed by ordinary metabolic breakdown of organic compounds. In other words, from digestion of food, from muscle exertion and other body activity. The body defenses can handle some of these free devils because it developed procedures long ago.   The body manufactures a complex system of antioxidant chemicals and antioxidant enzymes. They include enzymes such as superoxide dismutase, catalase, and glutathione peroxidase. The antioxidant chemicals include vitamins A, C, E, and Beta-carotene, the minerals selenium and zinc, and the amino acids cysteine and methionine.

Because we live in a polluted atmosphere, it is doubtful that the body can receive sufficient nutrients from the food we eat to satisfy the normal metabolic needs and its antioxidant needs. For example, when the trace mineral selenium meets with the harmful metal mercury in the body and combines with it to remove it from the body, there may not be sufficient selenium remaining to meet other selenium needs. Providing the essential nutrients as supplements allows for the proper function of the antioxidant defense system.

Although many nutrients have antioxidant functions, those most frequently recognized as having outstanding capacity are vitamin C, vitamin E, selenium and Beta-carotene.

Vitamin E may be the supreme oxygen efficiency nutrient. In all of its biological functions, vitamin E has been shown to behave as both a protective antioxidant against free radical activity and as an oxygen conservator for needed body use of oxygen. According to Dr. Robert Tengerdy, world expert on vitamin E at Colorado State University, proper immune function may require six times the vitamin E previously thought to be nutritionally adequate.

At an international meeting in Kyoto, Japan in April of 1988, 750 scientists described dozens of studies in animals and people demonstrating the potential benefits of anti-free radical therapy in a wide spectrum of disorders from influenza to heart attacks. Among the mentioned substances already in general use are, for example, nutrients like vitamin E and Beta-carotene which are naturally present in foods and vitamin C, both naturally present and added to some foods, which work by countering free radical formation or by "mopping up" free radicals as they form.

It seems hopeless to prevent free radical formation. Many factors initiate radical production, most are uncontrollable like heat, radiation, heavy exercise, inflammation, air pollution, tobacco smoke, pesticides, asbestos, phenobarbital, certain anticancer drugs, cured meats, dietary fats, sunlight . . . and on and on. But, we can use our heads and not smoke, protect ourselves from the U.V. rays of the sun, even drink filtered water. Still, the best protection appears to be to support the systems nature has provided. We can take supplements of the various substances the diet cannot provide in the needed amounts to neutralize the environment.

For example, animal studies have shown that vitamin E can help protect against ozone-induced free radical damage. This can be especially severe in areas like the Los Angeles basin where the ozone content of smog can reach ten or more times the usual amount of ozone at sea level.

Superoxide dismutase and catalase and glutathione peroxidase help convert free radicals to less toxic substances like water. In fact, one type of therapy now under study at Duke University, of animals exposed to lung-damaging free radicals, uses fatty capsules containing SOD (superoxide dismutase) and catalase to prolong their lives. A similar approach might be useful in emphysema patients to limit the extent of lung injury.

Natural Free Radical Scavengers

Because vitamin E is a fat soluble vitamin it can penetrate fatty cell membranes and remove the unpaired electron from a free radical before it causes damage. This "scavenging" effect converts the free radical into a less reactive substance.

Vitamin C, being water soluble, can perform the same task in a watery medium and can help regenerate vitamin E to its active scavenger form. Beta-carotene (a substance found in carrots and dark green leafy vegetables and converted by the body into vitamin A), protects the body against free radicals and also uric acid.

Selenium increases the activity and retention of vitamin E in the body. Its antioxidant activity is directly related to glutathione peroxidase formation since each molecule of glutathione contains four atoms of selenium. As a component of this enzyme, selenium protects cell membrane, helps prevent cardiovascular disease, helps reduce the incidence of cancer and is imperative to the control of chemical hypersensitivity. Likewise it strengthens the immune system, helps increase normal energy levels and can slow down the aging process.

How Much of the Supplements Do We Need?

There are a number of antioxidant formulas available in health food stores and in drugstores. Most of them have adequate amounts of the nutrients. Since we are all individuals and all eat different diets, no one formula is ideal for all. Selenium is a trace mineral and its bodily needs are measured in micrograms. The National Research Council has recommended a daily intake of 50 to 200 micrograms. Two of the world's most noted selenium authorities, Drs. Schrauzer and Shamberger suggest that the daily adult intake should equal 250 to 350 mcgs. Since selenium is possibly toxic in doses over 450 mcgs. a day, doses over the recommended amount should not be used without a doctor's supervision.

Vitamin C is also an antioxidant, immunity enhancer and a protector against aging. In doses of 1 to 3 grams daily, vitamin C is said to stimulate the immune system, help decrease blood cholesterol levels, and fight off free radicals. Vitamin C is excreted from the blood within 4 or so hours, so in order to maintain maximum blood levels, at least 200 milligrams must be taken four times a day. Or, get a good time-disintegrating formula that will last 8 to 10 hours.

Vitamin E, in doses of from 400 International Units to 1,000 I.U. may be the best of the free radical fighters. All good formulas will contain vitamin E.

Although not in all formulas, L-cysteine (an amino acid) helps protect against radiation damage, damage from smoking and drinking. If you take L-cysteine, make sure to take at least twice the amount of vitamin C with it.

Zinc, vitamin A, Beta-carotene are antioxidants and also synergists to the other free radical fighters. They also act against heavy metal poisons from automobile exhaust.

A complete protection program will have to include other nutrients besides the suggested antioxidants. The B-vitamins plus the minerals manganese and copper are important.

According to *FASEB Journal* 1:441-445 (1987). Clinical Nutrition, Hoffmann-La Roche. Lawrence J. Machlin and Adrianne Bendich, "Free radical tissue damage: protective role of antioxidant nutrients."

"Low levels of the antioxidant nutrients have been correlated with disease risk for cancer at several sites and for heart disease. Cataracts, inflammatory diseases such as arthritis, and the aging process itself have all been associated with free radical damage."

Broccoli

According to *Science News*, April, 1985, broccoli is one of the best natural antioxidants you can eat. It may increase your glutathione activity. There is a chemical in broccoli and in other cruciferous vegetables such as cabbage and cauliflower that are helpful in washing harmful substances out of the body or in helping to counteract their harmful activity.

Seaweed

One of the better ways to help remove metal traces from your body is with seaweed. Seaweed contains sodium alginate which combines with toxic substances and helps remove them from the body through the waste mechanism.

Chlorella

Can be part of a detoxification process to get rid of accumulated waste material. (See later section on Chlorella.)

Garlic and Lead Poisoning

Garlic helps prevent the peroxidation of fatty acids and the formation of other free radical end products. Like other antioxidant substances, garlic exerts a protective effect against toxic heavy metals. The metals — lead, mercury and cadmium — are bound by garlic which then helps lead them from the body. In one Russian study, a preparation made from garlic extract was given to workers suffering from lead poisoning. Subsequent testing showed great improvement.

Garlic is also a natural source of germanium. Other plants which contain germanium are ginseng, comfrey and aloe, three plants noted for their healing powers.

Cholesterol From the Inside
and From the Outside

There are new findings about cholesterol.

They appear to indicate that it is only when cholesterol is oxidized that it is dangerous.

That makes sense because the *body naturally produces cholesterol* to help form the membranes of its cells and to provide an insulating sheath around nerve fibers. It also contributes to the manufacture of hormones and to the production of vitamin D.

April 3, 1989, University of Southern California news release: Watching cholesterol?

Maybe you should start watching cholesterol oxides.

Recent research suggests you can better protect yourself against atherosclerosis — heart-threatening clogging of the arteries — if you have your blood monitored for the oxide compounds produced when cholesterol is broken down in the body.

And . . . the way to lower your blood levels of cholesterol oxides is not only to limit your consumption of cholesterol from foods, not only to use garlic, onion, fish oil, phytosterols, etc. but *also to take antioxidants such as vitamin E!*

Dr. Alex Sevanian, Ph.D., an associate professor at the University of Southern California School of Pharmacy has said that laboratory studies confirm the growing scientific suspicion that the risk of atherosclerosis is determined much more accurately from the oxidation of blood lipids (fats) and, specifically, the levels of cholesterol oxides than from cholesterol itself.

"And we've developed laboratory evidence that blood levels of cholesterol oxides can be reduced with vitamin E."

The research appears to further indicate that cholesterol oxides may be the real culprits that trigger the formation of the plaque (fatty tissue) that clogs arteries.

Sevanian, in collaboration with David H. Blankenhorn, M.D., and Donald W. Crawford, M.D. of the USC School of Medicine's Atherosclerosis Research Institute has conducted a number of pioneering studies on cholesterol oxidation.

Using synthetic membrane systems, Sevanian and his colleagues have demonstrated that cholesterol is readily oxidized in the presence of other fatty compounds. They've homed in on the fact that there is no damage from cholesterol, but that cholesterol oxides are toxic, in the sense that they irritate and inflame endothelial cells.

Then they've demonstrated in animal studies that dietary supplements of vitamin E will reduce the body's production of cholesterol epoxide, the major by-product of cholesterol oxidation.

Sevanian, whose cholesterol research is funded by the National Institute of Health, says that the laboratory findings are sufficiently convincing to justify trials on human subjects.

That is not to say that taking vitamin E will enable you to ignore good dietary habits and let you eat all the fat and cholesterol containing foods that you want. You will still have to watch your intake, trim fats from meat, eat more fowl and fish, eat more fresh vegetables and whole grains, and use other supplements. There's so much fat in all of the fast food we eat that we need all the help we can get.

Grapefruit Pectin and Cholesterol

Cerda J. Robbins F. Burgin C, et al: "The Effects of Grapefruit Pectin on Patients at Risk for Coronary Heart Disease." *Clin. Card.* 1988;11:589-594.

Grapefruit pectin lowered plasma cholesterol levels 7.6% in a study conducted at the University of Florida College of Medicine.

27 people received either 15 grams of grapefruit pectin or a placebo in a 16 week crossover, double-blind study. No changes were made in the diet or the lifestyle.

In addition to lowering total cholesterol, the grapefruit pectin lowered bad cholesterol levels as well.

Guar Gum and Cholesterol

Ebeling P, Hannele Y, Antti A, et al: "The Effects of Guar Gum." *Am. J. Clin. Nutr.* 1988; 43:98-103.

Guar gum can reduce postprandial blood glucose and serum total cholesterol.

Granulated guar gum in 5 gram amounts taken 4 time a day before meals, reduced serum cholesterol 21% after four weeks of trial.

Guar gum and pectin are both available at health food stores and drug stores. They may be part of diet formulas and not sold as a treatment for high cholesterol content in the body.

Cholesterol Lowering Fibers

News about recent research on oat bran and its remarkable ability to lower serum cholesterol 15 to 20% has been sweeping the country.

Another popular dietary fiber is also as effective as oat bran. It's called psyllium husks. Dr. James Anderson at the University of Kentucky, has been working on oat bran and psyllium husks and has found both fibers to be equally effective in lowering elevated cholesterol levels.

Other fibers with cholesterol-lowering effects include barley, guar and pectin.

They also have other toxin-eliminating effects. This table illustrates some of the research findings on dietary fibers and their sources:

Oat bran
Guar gum
Pectin
Psyllium husks
* lower blood cholesterol levels

Psyllium husks
Barley fiber
Pectin
Wheat bran
* speeds transit time and helps detoxify the colon

Psyllium husks
Barley fiber
Wheat bran
Rice bran
* absorbs water in the colon, helps remove toxins and promotes easier elimination.

The Rutgers University *Guide to Lowering Cholesterol, Health Academy Series,* by Hans Fisher, Ph.D. and Eugene Boe deals with a number of means to help control your intake of possibly toxic cholesterol or even to block some of the dietary cholesterol from absorption. Dietary considerations include:

* limiting red meat consumption
* choosing lean cuts
* trimming away all visible fat
* avoiding processed or luncheon meats, sausage, bacon, liver and kidneys.
* eating more poultry without the skin, fish, dried beans and peas, tofu.
* having skim milk or low-fat milk and cheese.
* using butter sparingly.
* using less eggs.
* eating more plant foods and whole grains.

Also:
Increase your fiber intake.
Eat more fish (NOTE: It is the author's opinion that capsules of fish oil used as supplements fit more easily into the American style of eating. If you are not a fish lover, use capsules of Max Epa, two

capsules with each meal, available at health food stores or at drugstores.)

Eat more garlic and onions (AUTHOR'S NOTE: or take garlic and onions in capsule form. Even the deodorized garlic will benefit your body . . . and you won't be offensive.)

Get more plant sterols into your diet.

Plant sterols (phytosterols) are known to inhibit cholesterol absorption, perhaps by interfering in the exchange process necessary for the transport of cholesterol through the mucous lining.

Plant sterols such as beta-sitosterol and campesterol are fatty alcohols found in a wide variety of vegetables, grains and seeds, including eggplant, cabbage, peanuts, rice, yams, barley and avocados.

(AUTHOR'S NOTE: Phytosterols are also available in supplement form. If you take one or two tablets or capsules before meals, depending on the kind of meal you are eating, the ingredients can react with the cholesterol in the meal and help prevent a portion of the cholesterol from entering the bloodstream.)

How much is needed?

A daily intake of 300 milligrams of phytosterols (based on the beta-sitosterol content) has been shown to have a significant cholesterol-lowering effect.

"Effects of Chlorella on Levels of Cholesterol in Serum and Liver." From a team of researchers at the Wakahisa Hospital of Fukuoka where sixteen patients were given chlorella (20 tablets a day) for three months, without any anti-cholesterol drugs. The result was that their cholesterol levels dropped significantly.

American Journal of Clinical Nutrition, 1988;47:67-77

Drs. Zara D. Abraham and Tara Mehta, at the Department of Food Science and Human Nutrition of Washington State University gave seven men a controlled diet including psyllium husk. Ten days later and again in three weeks the scientists measured the blood cholesterol of their subjects and found reductions both in low-density and high-density cholesterol without decreases in nutrient absorption.

Get the Lead Out, and the Cadmium,
and the Mercury

In *Discover* magazine, May 1988 . . . think twice before taking a sip from a public water fountain.

A House subcommittee on Health and the Environment survey uncovered the previously unknown fact that millions of public drinking fountains, especially scuttlebutts in the military, are pouring harmful amounts of lead into the drinkers system.

Those shiny metal water fountains feature either lead-lined cooling tanks or lead solder, and these lead components leach concentrations of the heavy metal ranging from 30 parts per billion to 100 parts per billion.

Ron Levin, author of the EPA study on lead contamination of water, told the lawmakers that if a water fountain is producing 50 parts per billion or more, it should be pulled out. The EPA was alerted to the problem when it was found that two U.S. Navy fountains were giving off high concentrations of lead. One fountain unloaded 830 parts per billion.

Water fountains have a life span of 30 years and there are millions of them around the nation. This pollution has been going on for a long time and we can best counter it by getting rid of the offending fountains and using nutritionally active substances to help get the lead out.

Why all of the fuss?

Because lead accumulates in the body and in the brain. Mercury and lead combine to be even more toxic to our systems. Both metals are widespread pollutants. Dr. Kazuhiko Asai points out in his book *Organic Germanium, Miracle Cure*, that the oxidation-enhancing and "metal trapping" qualities of germanium has proved effective in helping Japanese victims of mercury toxicity. The germanium compound is discharged from the body along with some of the toxic material.

The usual dose for germanium is 150 milligrams a day in divided doses. It is available from health food stores and drugstores.

According to an article by Stephen A. Levine, Ph.D. which appeared in *Health World*, Summer, 1987, germanium enhances the oxygen supply to the tissues without increasing free radical damage. Since oxygen is essential to good health, it is necessary to be able to balance its beneficial effects against its damaging effects and germanium appears to be able to do that.

Radiation Protection

Radiation has always existed and life always had to cope with it. Radiation does harm to the body in three ways. It can directly strike and harm biological molecules. It can convert its energy into heat which "cooks" tissues. It can produce highly reactive free radicals.

The body has learned to cope with radiation to some extent in that it makes enzymes which can cool off the super-heated free radical. The enzyme which does a great deal of work in the body is SOD (superoxide dismutase).

When superoxide dismutase has done its work upon super-oxide, all that is left behind is oxygen and hydrogen peroxide. Hydrogen peroxide, if left alone, will eventually form hydroxyl radicals which could do damage in themselves. However, another enzyme, catalase, dismutes the hydrogen peroxide into water and oxygen.

Supplements of these enzymes are available in health food stores and drug stores. (*Health Express*, Dr. William Ellis, D.O. "Antioxidant Enzymes," April, 1982.)

Sea vegetables like kelp and dulse contain sodium alginate which are effective in removing free radical producing heavy metals from the body.

Miso contains zybicolin, which has properties similar to sodium alginate. Nori also contains zybicolin. ("Surviving Radiation," Zane Baranowski, *Health World*, Summer, 1987.)

Sea vegetables can be purchased at Health food stores.

Herbs Help Your Body Cleanse Itself

When potentially toxic substances such as insecticides, pesticides, herbicides, etc. are used on fruits and vegetables, even the most careful washing won't be able to get rid of all of it. Sometimes, substances like Alar — used on apples — penetrate the fruit and are impossible to remove.

Most of the toxins we ingest are in such small amounts that our stomachs do not reject them. We seem to have adjusted well enough to industrial poisons that we don't throw up, and the result is that toxins enter our digestive tracts day in and day out and are stored in the body cells.

Our bodies, in an attempt to manage these substances, try to excrete them through the urinary system. This doesn't mean that they can pass through the body without doing some damage. Many substances can have harmful effects on the kidneys, the bladder, etc., as they are passing through. If the toxic substances are not passed out in the urine, the body stores them in various places — the liver, the fat cells, the bones, the muscles, the digestive tract. A large amount of toxic material may be stored in the colon or large intestine.

Many herbs are able to stimulate a cleansing of the colon. Herbs such as cascara sagrada, black walnut, psyllium seed husks, fennel seed, fenugreek, slippery elm, etc. These herbs use gentle laxative action to promote cleansing.

Health food stores and drugstores carry a number of herbal formulas to stimulate healthful cleansing of toxic material. You can do other things to enhance the effect:

1) Remove as many toxin-containing foods from the diet as you possibly can.

2) If the water in your area is contaminated, purchase bottled water to drink and use in cooking.

3) Drink plenty of fluids every day to wash out toxins that can be eliminated through the urine and the feces.

4) Stay regular and avoid constipation.

Special colonic rinse formulas may have benefits in clearing out toxic material from the intestinal walls. They are a selected mix of herbs designed to remove plaque, excess mucus, and toxins. If this can be accomplished, there will be better absorption of nutrients into the bloodstream. Herbs and minerals (bentonite, wheatgrass, citrus pectin, psyllium husks, cascara sagrada, diatomacious earth, chamomile and lactobacillus acidophilus) are all combined in a colonic "wash."

Although this is not the only combination formula on the market and there are many good formulas, it is an example of the synergism to be expected when you purchase a colon cleanser. Your health food store can show you a number of food cleansers. Follow label instructions.

Ginseng and Stress

The adverse effects of drugs, food additives, environmental chemicals and other pollutants can cause a number of stress-related problems. People complain of general fatigue, cold hands and feet, backache, insomnia, depression and digestive problems.

While the Koreans were primarily responsible for introducing Americans to ginseng in the 1950's and 60's — they use it daily as a general health tonic, mostly as a tea — other Asian countries combine it with other herbs to enhance its effects.

Stress is a term which effectively sums up a wide range of many adverse effects on our general health. The physical and biological, emotional and dietary pressures can cause a weakening of the immune system and the loss of overall energy — especially when pollutants become toxic and build up in the body. Ginseng, by itself or in combination with other herbs, has been shown to be highly effective in guarding against the health-depleting effects of stress.

Here are some formulas which can be purchased in health food stores:

A combination of Ginseng, Licorice, Holen, Atractylodes
A combination of Ginseng, Tang-Kuei, Peony, Rehmannia
A combination of Ginseng, Astragalus, Schizandra
A combination of Ginseng, Citrus

The labels will give you instructions and indicate the use of each combination.

Detoxicants — a Variety of Ways

Perhaps the most clearly observable effect of garlic is its detoxifying effect on the body. It neutralizes toxins present in the digestive tract and eliminative organs as well as in the blood.

Onions, marjoram, and green chilies also possess an antioxidant effect and have been used for centuries for this beneficial action.

Lead, mercury, cadmium, arsenic and copper poisoning are becoming epidemic. Lead and mercury come mostly from polluted air plus industrial and medical uses such as lead-contaminated paint and mercury-containing amalgam dental fillings. Contaminated fish are also a source of mercury poisoning. Copper usually enters our bodies from copper water pipes.

Heavy metal poisoning is difficult to treat. Now, a Japanese study conducted by Drs. Ikezoe and Kitahara shows that a raw garlic extract developed in Japan and called Kyolic is protective against the effects of heavy metal poisoning.

Medical Journal, *Kiṣo-to-Rinsho*, Japan, March 1975.

In another study conducted in Russia, a drug made from garlic extract was given to workers in industrial plants who were suffering from chronic lead poisoning. The daily doses of garlic improved the symptoms of lead poisoning.

Petrov, V. et al. Gigiena Truda I. Prof. Zabolevaniya, 9(4), 42, 1955.

Dr. Constance Kies from the University of Nebraska, has found that psyllium husk fiber has positive effects on gastrointestinal function and is a detoxifier, helping to reduce gastrointestinal toxicity and also the absorption of cholesterol.

The soluble fibers in psyllium husks, guar and pectin have more positive effects than other plant fibers including wheat bran.

They are also able to bind heavy toxic metals, including lead and cadmium, in the gut and remove them from the body.

Bland, J. *Intestinal Toxicity and Inner Cleansing*, Keats Pub., New Canaan, Conn. 1987.

Spirulina, a green algae, has been used in Japan to treat victims of heavy metal poisoning, particularly that of cadmium. When spirulina has been ingested there has been an increased excretion of some contaminants.

Spirulina by J. J. Challem, Keats Pub., New Canaan, Conn., 1981.

Cigarettes Contain:
Carbon monoxide
Nitrogen oxide
Lead
Arsenic
Radioactive polonium
Nicotine
and more carcinogens . . .

If you smoke or are exposed to cigarette smoke, take the following nutrients as basic protection:

Vitamin A	10,000 I.U.
Vitamin E	1,000 I.U.
Vitamin C	3,000 mg
Vitamin B-1	50 mg
Vitamin B-3	50 mg
Pantothenic Acid	50 mg
B-6	50 mg
PABA	50 mg
Selenium	200 mcg
Zinc	25 mg
L-Cysteine	500 mg

International Institute of Health Sciences, Huntington Beach, CA., 1980.

Quick Reference for some of the nutrients destroyed by poisons in our environment:

POISON	WHAT'S LOST
Air pollutants	all vitamins
Alcohol	vitamins A, D, B-Complex, magnesium
Arsenic	PABA, A
Carbon monoxide	vitamin C
Chlorine	vitamin E
Caffeine	vitamin B-complex, potassium, zinc
Nitrates/Nitrites	vitamins, A, C, E

What do do?

Take a good nutritional supplement since you can't avoid everything . . .

Lipoic Acid

Chemically, lipoic acid is classified as a coenzyme, meaning it is an essential component of an enzyme. Although it has many properties similar to a vitamin it is not essential — meaning that it can be manufactured in the body. However, as part of a formula, lipoic acid is able to induce the body to use unwanted waste material as fuel for energy thereby ridding the body of this material.

Carnitine, another fat-burning nutrient, works fairly simply by transferring fats into the little engine that powers every cell in the body. Then the engine (called the mitochondria) burns up the fat. Lipoic acid follows more complex metabolic pathways. In technical terms, lipoic acid works to move byproducts to the Krebs' cycle by helping to breakdown and metabolize what is known as pyruvate, resulting in the production of ATP (adenosine triphosphate). ATP, sometimes called the universal energy component, is responsible for muscle contraction, the transportation of minerals and other nutrients, and other important functions.

Although it has been studied because of its interest to sprinters and others who require quick bursts of energy, recent evidence reveals that it has preventive and therapeutic use as well, particularly in regard to poisoning by such metals as lead, arsenic and mercury. Animal studies have shown that lipoic acid may even have cholesterol-lowering capabilities.

It is usually found combined with other nutrients in health food stores. Follow label instructions.

Weber, M.M., "Selenium Prevents the Growth-stimulating Effects of Cadmium on the Human Prostate Epithelium." *Biochem. Biophy. Res. Commun.* 127930:871-877, 1985

While cadmium was found to stimulate the growth of human prostatic epithelium, (at proper concentrations) selenium inhibited this action.

Korpela, H. et al. *Am. J. Clin. Nutr.* 42:147-151, 1985

Selenium: essential for the activity of glutathione peroxidase which protects against alcohol-induced liver damage.

Serum selenium was evaluated in 46 alcoholics and was found to be lower than in healthy controls. Its level was related to the severity of the liver disease and was lowest in those with de-compensated alcoholic cirrhosis.

Vitamin B-6 and MSG

Folkers, K. et al. "Biochemical Evidence for a Deficiency of Vitamin B-6 in Subjects Reacting to Monosodium-L-Glutamate by the Chinese Restaurant Syndrome." (*Biochem. Biophys. Res. Commun.* 100:972-7, 1981.

Supplemental use of vitamin B-6 may be helpful for those people sensitive to MSG. The dosage was 50 mg. daily.

Subjects sensitive to MSG were given vitamin B-6 supplements for 12 weeks and then subjected to MSG. Most of the subjects showed no response to MSG.

Phytosterols

Mattson, F.H. et al. "Optimizing the Effect of Plant Sterols on Cholesterol Absorption by as much as 64% in Man." *Am. J. Clin. Nutr.* 35:697-700, 1982.

The title says it all. 300 mg of phytosterols daily (based on beta-sitosterol content) immediately before or after a meal decreased cholesterol absorption by as much as 64%.

And . . . may even wash serum cholesterol out of the body.

Beveridge et al. *Can. J. Biochem. Physiol.* 36:895, 1958.

May reduce serum cholesterol even in the total absence of dietary cholesterol.

Eggplant with vitamin C

Mitschek, GHA. *Experimentelle Pathalogie*, Vol. 10, 1975.

Animals fed eggplant along with vitamin C rich foods were protected from developing fatty plaques.

Garlic and Onions

Ernst, E. et al. "Garlic and Blood Lipid Levels." *Brit. Med. J.* 291:139, 1985.

Ten patients were treated with 600 mg garlic powder daily (equivalent to 1800 gm fresh garlic) and showed a 10% decrease in cholesterol levels and triglyceride levels.

Atherosclerosis 26:379-82, 1977.

The administration of garlic and onion prevented the formation of experimental atherosclerosis in rabbits.

Cooking with Ginger

Nutr. Rep. Int. 17:183-9, 1978.

"Effect of Ginger on Serum and Hepatic Cholesterol Levels in Cholesterol Fed Rats." Gujaral S. et al.

It appears that the use of ginger as a supplement may reduce cholesterol levels.

Vitamin C, E, and Nitrosamines

The antioxidant vitamins C and E may help prevent nitrates and nitrites in smoked, pickled or cured foods from being converted in the body to nitrosamines which have been linked to cancer of the stomach and the esophagus.

National Academy of Science, Nutrition, Diet and Cancer, 1982. *Complementary Medicine*, Vol. 3, No. 1, 1987

In the U.S., the Environmental Protection Agency has identified more than 700 regularly occurring pollutants in drinking water. Of those that have now been tested, 22 are known to cause cancer.

The most common pollutants are the trihalomethanes (THM's) including chloroform, tetrachloride, tetrachloroethylene, and trichloroethane, which are present in virtually all chlorinated water in the United States. Chloroform can cause liver and kidney damage and central nervous system depression.

Am. J. Epidem., 126:772, 1987. "Smoking and Beta-Carotene."

The association between diet and cigarette use on plasma Beta-carotene levels was assessed at Channing Laboratory in Boston.

Men who smoked one pack a day had only 72% of the plasma Beta-carotene levels of nonsmokers, even with normal dietary intake.

Prescription Drug News, Vol. 2, No. 7, 1987

Cancerous tumors in the mouth can be reduced or prevented by carotene, according to researchers at Harvard University. Carotene is a natural substance found in fruits and vegetables which is turned into vitamin A in the body.

According to the study published in *Carcinogenesis*, cancerous tumors in hamsters' mouths disappeared within two weeks after the Beta-carotene solution had been applied directly onto the tumors or injected into the mouth.

Mutat. Res. 1988;199:85-93

Francis, A., Shetty, T., Bhattach, R: "Modifying Role of Dietary Factors on the Mutagenicity of Aflatoxin B: In Vitro Effects of Trace Elements."

There was great alarm raised when it was discovered that corn and other grains had a higher than average amount of a toxic substance called aflatoxin. As a result of the lack of rain, the corn became less resistant to the mold Aspergillus flavus. Much of the corn was considered to be too dangerous to feed to humans since aflatoxins are both mutagenic and carcinogenic. They produce liver cancer in several animal species and are a suspected human carcinogen.

Since it was considered too dangerous to feed to humans, the "correct" agencies decided it was okay to feed to animals what would then be fed to humans . . .

However, researchers at the Bhabha Atomic Research Center in Bombay, India have discovered that the trace elements copper, manganese, zinc, and selenium all exhibit ability to inhibit the mutagenesis induced by aflatoxin.

Past research has shown that vitamins (most notably vitamin B-2, retinoids, trace metals, fatty acids, and flavonoids) can act against these contaminants.

Hans Nieper, M.D., Phoenix, Arizona, 1986

Squalene is obtained from the liver of the Aizame shark. They are found swimming in icy cold water at depths of 3,000 feet off the islands of Okinawa.

When squalene is given to a patient, we first see that he is more resistant to developing herpes virus infections, for example, and far more resistant to developing cervical carcinoma or to developing positive pap tests. Squalene requires tremendous amounts of ascorbate to be converted to its active form. As a result, we have given vitamin C in higher doses together with squalene. Then the endogenous production of repair substances which work both against the virus and the cancer cell genome is highly enhanced. Now this justifies Linus Pauling who pointed out that high doses of vitamin C seemed to do something in cancer patients . . . and he is absolutely right. What he didn't know is that vitamin C is only activated (by) higher concentrations of such repair substances, for instance, once you give the precursor squalene.

(Some health food stores carry squalene for internal and external use. Squalene may also be obtained from olive oil so there's no need to kill the sharks.)

Squalene, as a moisturizing agent, helps protect the skin against smoke and pollution.

Old Herbs, Mushrooms & Chlorella

Herbs have been around before there were people, and ever since people found out about herbs' usefulness they have been used as food and medicine.

Ginkgo biloba is the oldest known tree genus. These trees have been around since the dinosaur roamed the earth. They survived the Ice Age and can even live amid the fumes from cars' exhausts. Although there is no cure for old age and the problems associated with poor circulation, there may be at least partial relief with preparations derived from the leaves of this ancient plant. It appears that Ginkgo extracts help increase the flow of nutrients and oxygen to the body's extremities. When poor circulation or pollution has interfered with mental abilities causing a loss in mental alertness, Ginkgo has the unique ability to "tune up" the thinking machine.

Milk thistle, Silybum marianum, is an herb that specifically protects the liver. The liver is the detoxifying plant in the body. It acts against many poisons, rendering them harmless or excreting them through the kidneys. However, if the liver is scarred or sick, it can't do the job and the toxic elements can overwhelm the body.

The milk thistle, the scourge of farmers, a disagreeable and pesty weed, has now been determined to yield a compound that helps protect and heal the liver from a number of toxins and toxic effects.

Benda, L., Dittrich, H., Ferenzi, P., Frank, H., and Wewalks, F. "The Influence of Therapy with Sylymarin on the Survival Rate of Patients with Liver Cirrhosis." *Wiener Klinische Wodenschrift*, Oct. 10, 1980, p. 678.

A double-blind study on the therapy of patients with alcoholic liver cirrhosis shows a significantly higher survival rate in the group treated with silymarin. This result can be explained by the ability of this substance to protect the liver against toxic injuries.

It was only a matter of time before modern science, particularly in Germany, began to examine the folk lore claims made for this herb. Now there is sufficient research (some 200 papers have been published) to say that the herb does protect and help regenerate the liver.

Magliulo, E., Carosi, P.G., Minoli, L., and Corini, S. "Studies on the Regenerative Capacity of the Liver in Rats Subjected to Partial Hepatectomy and Treated with Silymarin." Arzneim-Forsch (*Drug Res.*) 1973, 23, Nr. la. p. 161.

Studies were performed to examine whether a single protective dose of i.v. injected silymarin was able to modify, in partially hepatectomized rats, the rate of liver regeneration as well as the intrinsic reproductive activity of the liver cells. The results obtained provided statistically significant evidence that silymarin speeds up the regeneration process and heightens the mitotic rate of regeneration of liver cells.

No side effects from the use of milk thistle have been observed when used to treat deadly mushroom poisoning such as from amanita. In the 1970's in Europe, 60 patients with mushroom poisoning were treated with a special extract of milk thistle. They all survived, when the normal death rate would have been 30 to 40 percent.

Silymarin, the chief constituent of milk thistle, is currently listed in the *Merck Index*, the bible of conventional medicine in the U.S., as a protectant for the liver.

Milk thistle is also one of the only known substances that can protect the liver against damage by some environmental pollutants. Clincial stresses on the liver are widespread in modern society. Any dysfunction in the liver, even if not manifesting an overt disease, is felt profoundly. Subclinical syndromes may include low energy, sleepiness after meals, irritability, headaches, depression, poor digestion and even acne. Milk thistle has no known toxicity and mice love it as a food and thrive on it.

Tablets and capsules of silymarin are available in health food stores. Follow label directions.

Echinacea: Good for What Ails You

Especially if it's a cold or the flu. Echinacea has become increasing popular as an immune stimulant as pollution increases. It strengthens the body, enabling it to fight off a myriad of ailments. It is not appropriate for long term use but is very effective at the onset of a cold or the flu.

Astragalus: Chinese Immune Enhancer

Astragalus combinations have been used in traditional Chinese medicine to re-energize those people who are debilitated and weak. It has been tried against AIDS at the Quan Yin Clinic in San Francisco.

Chlorella

This is a green, single-celled microalgae, about two and a half billion years old, containing more chlorophyll than any other organism on earth. It is a substance necessary for detoxification and is also an aid to the entire digestive process.

It is available in a number of forms in health food stores. Follow label directions.

Reishi Mushrooms

This mushroom grows on plum trees and has a history of medicinal value that goes back over 2,000 years.

Shitake Mushrooms

This is a flesh mushroom produced under controlled growing conditions. Like the Reishi mushroom, the Shitake contains a substance called *lentinan* in high concentrations. Both mushrooms exhibit the ability to influence vitality and life-prolonging properties.

According to researchers at Kobe University in Japan, the mushrooms produce interferon and the interferon helps to fight invading bacterial pollutants.

Mushrooms are available in tablet form in most health food stores. Follow label directions.

Suma (Pfaffia Paniculata)

From deep within the Amazon's rain forest comes one of the amazing herbs. The Indians call it "Para toda" meaning for all things because of its many applications. It has been used in the Amazon for at least three hundred years for its ability to cure skin problems caused by pollutants.

It is available in the U.S. in health food stores. Follow label directions.

Gallus Domesticus

Lastly, the power of a hot water infusion of selected parts of the Gallus domesticus . . . the common chicken.

Chicken soup has long been recognized as an important part of the doctor's armamentarium. As early as the 12th Century, the physician Moses Maimonides wrote, "chicken soup . . . is recommended as an excellent food as well as medication." He further specified that one should "not use the too large, that is more than 2 years of age; not the too small, that is those in whom the mucus still prevails; neither the too lean, nor those who through feeding become obese; but those that are fat by nature, without being stuffed."

Rosner, F. and Munter, S., *The Medical Writings of Maimonides*, Lippincott, Philadelphia, 1969.

Chicken soup was used in Europe for centuries, but disappeared from commercial production after the inquisition. It remained popular in European tradition and its use has grown steadily over the last three hundred years.

While details of the chemistry of chicken soup are poorly understood, it is recognized that the composition of this material can vary considerably. It has been shown that one of the properties of chicken soup is to hasten the removal of pathogens from the nose. It appears to be an effective adjunct in the treatment of mild upper respiratory tract infections.

Pollution and Your Hair

Nutrition plays a very important part in the health of your hair. Protein, vitamin B-Complex — especially pantothenic acid and biotin — vitamin E, and a good diet, plenty of water and exercise. But pollutants can rob your hair of its looks and strength. Pollutants get in your hair and it takes a good shampoo to get hair clean.

A good shampoo should be gentle enough to use every day, yet it should clean your hair of unwanted contaminants, dirt, styling gel, grime, smog, and whatever else is floating in the air that day. But, unless your hair is ultra-oily, too-frequent shampooing can lead to dryness. Soaps tend to leave a drying and dulling film on your hair. That's true even of castile soap, so soap is best avoided if you want to keep your hair and promote its beauty. However, you can try soap substitutes such as sodium laureth sulfate, cocamidopropyl betaine, palm kernelamide, DEA, and coconut diethylnolamide. All of these are derived from coconuts and they contain ingredients to clean your hair gently.

Oil glands resting lovingly in your scalp secrete natural oils to keep your scalp pliant and free of flakes. Too often, however, internal conditions and external pollutants interfere with the amount of oil secreted. Hair conditioners are basically the secret to keeping your hair manageable and looking its best. After shampooing, hair has a negative electrical charge running through each strand. The drier the climate, the more electricity. One strand then acts to repel the other. With each hair acting negatively, the result is a head full of independent fibers or, "the fly-aways." A good conditioner will give your hair a positive charge and make it more manageable.

If you find a good shampoo and good conditioner . . . don't stick to them. Find two or three and alternate them every two or three weeks. This prevents your hair from getting used to the ingredients and keeps your hair alive and vital.

Perfect Solutions

When choosing your hair care routine, you'll get the best results when your shampoo and conditioner share the same active ingredients. Here's a guide:

Aloe Vera: Great for all types of hair, especially normal to oily. Its high zinc content is highly compatible with the hair's zinc-based structure. It also has an astringent action, tightening scalp pores that secrete excess oil and smoothing the hair to a lustrous shine.

Amino Acids: Your body relies on 22 amino acids to build proteins — and your hair is made of proteins. Amino acids also act to keep the hair pliant, soft and super-manageable.

Biotin: A member of the B-vitamin family, biotin is helpful in solving such common problems as falling hair, dry itchy scalp, and hair damage such as split ends.

Collagen Protein: Unlike Keratin protein (see below), Collagen protein makes hair more pliant by binding essential moisture to the hair's inner structure.

Dex-panthenol: This extra-strength form of pantothenol, the pro-vitamin of B-6, is one of the strongest moisture binders for hair care. It is excellent for hair that is super-dry, or damaged from perms, colorants or other special treatments.

Gingko Biloba: The powerful nutrients in the leaves of this tree will fight free radicals and stimulate your scalp to produce thicker, shinier, healthier hair.

Jojoba Oil: This is great for both oily and dry hair! The secret is its deepdown cleansing action that keeps dandruff, itching and hair loss at bay.

Keratin Protein: Once regarded as just a coating for hair, today's keratin proteins actually penetrate each hair strand, resulting in thicker, shinier hair. It also helps to repair split ends.

Tea Tree Oil: From the melaleuca tree, also called "Aussie Gold," this is another oil that is equally beneficial for oily, normal, or dry hair. It helps to make the hair extra-clean and extra-moist. Also, an anti-fungal component of Tea Tree Oil is effective against itchy, flaking scalp.

Nutritional Wandering Among World Literature

Some of the ways nutrients in food protect us:

The human body will try to select the raw material that is best for it. If it has a choice, it will take quality. However, if it happens to be offered a choice of something that is a pollutant but looks like a nutrient or nothing at all . . . it will settle for the pollutant and try to use it.

Strontium 90, the dangerous radioactive isotope, looks like calcium to the body. If it takes in strontium 90, it will try to use it like it uses calcium, store it in the teeth and the long bones. But it isn't calcium and can't do calcium's jobs in the body. We're not the only ones that get fooled. Plants and animals also take in strontium 90 and store it.

What's one of the answers?

Give your body calcium! If you supply adequate amounts of calcium the body will not pick up the strontium 90 and store it away. It will choose quality all of the time.

Will it work with other radioactive elements?

You can bet your life it will.

Cesium 137 is stored in the liver, the reproductive organs, muscles and kidneys. Potassium helps prevent body pick-up.

Cobalt 60 is stored in the liver and reproductive organs. Vitamin B-12 helps prevent body pick-up.

Iodine 131 is stored in the thyroid gland and the reproductive organs. Iodine helps prevent the body from storing it.

Sulfur 35 is stored in the skin. Sulfur helps get rid of it.

Zinc 65 is stored in the bones, but dietary zinc guards against it.

Also, remember that sea vegetables contain sodium alginate. When it meets substances like radioactive strontium it chelates (binds to them) to form a gel-like substance that leaves the body with the waste material.

Research has shown that sodium alginate can be used as both a preventive and therapeutic agent.

Tanka, Y., Stara, J. et al. "Application of Algal Polysaccharides as in Vivo Binders of Metal Pollutants," *Proceedings of the Seventh International Seaweed Symposium*, Aug. 8-12, 1971, John Wiley & Sons, 1971, p. 603.

Sodium alginate is found in sea vegetables such as arame, wakame, kombu, hijiki, and dulse. Dulse is the first one to try since it is closest to the American taste.

According to studies done by Tanaka and other scientists at McGill University, Gastro-Intestinal Research Laboratory in Montreal, sodium alginate is one of the prime protectives against environmental contaminants.

The United States Atomic Energy Commission has recognized the efficiency of sodium alginate. According to the Division of Biomedical and Environmental Research of the A.E.C., protection against radioactive poisoning for humans requires taking a minimum of two or three ounces of sea vegetables a week or ten grams (two tablespoons) a day of an alginate supplement.

If taken as a supplement, alginate in tablets or powder is more effective when mixed with enough fluid to make a gelatinous substance.

Some sea vegetables are a good source of iodine. Other food sources include Swiss chard, turnip greens, garlic, onions, mustard greens, asparagus, kale, seafoods, eggs and spinach — unless the soil is deficient in the mineral itself.

Which Nutrients Can Affect Which Pollutants?

According to the best literature, there are several natural substances which can be protective against pollutants. The following should be able to help you in your war:

Pollutant	Natural Substance
Aluminum	vitamin C
	zinc
	calcium
	magnesium
	lecithin
	fiber
Cadmium	cruciferous vegetables
	vitamin C
	vitamin D
	selenium
	manganese
	calcium
	copper
	pectin
	fiber
Carbon Monoxide	L-cysteine
	bee pollen
	nutritional yeast
	eleuthero
	vitamins A, B-Complex, C, E
Industrial Chemicals	bee pollen
	fermented foods
	all vitamins
	lecithin

Lead	pectin
	lecithin
	L-cysteine
	iron
	chlorophyll
	eleuthero
	phosphorous
	beans
	legumes
	cruciferous vegetables
	selenium
	sodium alginate
	all vitamins
	zinc
Mercury	cruciferous vegetables
	all vitamins
	L-cysteine
	selenium
	calcium
	fiber
	lecithin
	pectin
	nutritional yeast
Tobacco Smoke	selenium
	vitamin A, E, C
	zinc
	bee pollen
Smog	ginseng
	Vitamins A, C, B-Complex, E

Fermented Foods

Fermented foods have a beneficial effect on the intestines and help counteract toxins. They stimulate the production of friendly bacteria which live in the intestines. They promote healthy digestion and assimilation of nutrients. They also help detoxify the body. Yogurt is a good fermented food as is miso, tempeh, tamari, shoyu, and sauerkraut.

Nutritional Yeast

Grown expressly for human consumption, Saccharomyces cerevisiae, is a high-powered and concentrated food that can be protective against environmental pollutants.

Yeast has also been shown to reduce cholesterol levels and, according to Walter Mertz, Ph.D., Director of the Department of Agriculture's Human Nutrition Center, it helps normalize glucose utilization and blood sugar levels.

FROM FOLKLORE
TO SCIENCE

CONCENTRATED
HEALING FOODS

77 Scientific Adventures into the Power of
Herbs & Common Nutrients and the Astounding
Results of their Investigations as Reported
in the Nation's Important Journals.

by Dr. William H. Lee

FROM FOLKLORE TO SCIENCE

Since early Neanderthal man, plants have been used for healing. Throughout the centuries, while different modes of healing were tried, modified, discarded and then tried again, plants remained as the mainstay of medicine. Most of the plant remedies were discovered on a hit or miss basis. If they worked, they were remembered and passed on from generation to generation. Grandmothers passed their knowledge on to their daughters who passed it on to their daughters and so on. The knowledge became known as "Old Wives Tales," and then as "Folk Medicine."

For the most part, modern medicine ignored the wealth of plant medicine as old fashioned. At least they did until the holistic movement began to gain strength. People began to ask about the side effects of the potent drugs they were taking and why and what was the cause of their condition.

As more people began to ask questions, scientists themselves began to question modern medicine and began to look backwards in an effort to go forward. As they looked they discovered that there could be truth in some of the "Old Wives Tales."

Most writing concerned with herbology talks to the reader in anecdotes. This herb worked on such and such and I know it's true because my Aunt Susie had the same condition and it worked on her. This is the way "Folk Medicine" is usually taught and most of the anecdotes are true. However, this chapter goes beyond anecdotes. It describes actual scientific investigation and results!

You want to know if plants and nutrients can be effective medicines? Read on . . .

Applied and Environmental Microbiology, 36: 798-801.
Konowalchuk, J. and Speirs, J.I., "Antiviral Effects of Apple Beverages."

Freshly prepared apple juice has a powerful antiviral action against such crippling viruses as polio. The essential components which have this antiviral activity are located both in the skin and in the pulp of the apple.

Storage and/or exposure to heat will bring about a dramatic reduction in the apples ability to fight viruses.

Fresh grapes and fresh grape juice will also effectively destroy killer viruses. Apple cider and wine were less effective and the commercial apple drinks had no effect on them at all.

Journal of Pharmaceutical Sciences, 57: 1731, Oct. 1968. Bhargava, B.A., Westfall, U.C., and Siehr, D.J.,.Preliminary Pharmacology of Ellagic Acid from Juglans nigra (Black Walnut).

There are very few drugs that the physician can employ in cases of electrical shocks, accidental electrocution and lightening mishaps.

The Black Walnut, which has been used for centuries as a treatment for internal parasites, infection, tonsillitis, and has been used externally as an antiseptic, contains, as one of its active ingredients, a substance called ellagic acid.

Clinical experimentation within the last ten years has discovered that it is an ideal protective antidote for electrical mishaps.

Well-Being, Issue 34, p. 22, 1978. Nebelkopf, E., "The Healing Cacti."

The prickly pear (Opuntia species) is used by the natives against the bite of the tarantula. The pulp from a slashed leaf of this cacti, applied as a poultice to the bite will relieve the intense pain and swelling in a short time. However, few of us will have the misfortune to cross paths with an irritable tarantula. But, there seems to be another use for the nopal pads of the prickly pear that may be applicable for a larger number of people.

They are supposed to contain a large amount of natural organic insulin which will help the body to strengthen the pancreas and help to overcome diabetes.

Journal of the American Medical Association, 219:626.

An A.M.A. nutritionist has recommended chamomile as a delicious substitute for coffee for people with peptic ulcers, hypertension, heart problems, or anyone else who can no longer tolerate caffeine.

Journal of Clinical Pharmacology, Nov.-Dec. 1973.

Chamomile contains the amino acid tryptophan, which works like a sedative in the body, and will induce sleepiness much as warm milk would. When drugs failed, doctors gave heart patients this herb as a tea to help them sleep. Ten out of the twelve fell immediately into a deep slumber.

Journal of Agricultural and Food Chemistry, 23:943-49, 1975. Kaiser, R. et al, "Analysis of Buchu Leaf Oil."

Doctors frequently use diuretics (substances that can stimulate the flow of urine) to lessen edema or fluid accumulation in the body. Herbalists have used a combination of Buchu and Uva Ursi for the same reason for centuries.

Buchu contains an essential oil called pulegone which is also an antiseptic to the kidneys and valuable for any type of infection that affects that part of the body.

Well-Being, Issue 34, p. 22, 1978. Nebelkopf, E., "The Healing Cacti."

The night-blooming or sweet-scented cactus, biologically known as *Cactus grandiflorus* of the Cactaceae species grows in Jamaica. It has been used in folk medicine as a substitute for the heart stimulant — digitalis.

According to *Potter's Cyclopedia of Medicinal Herbs*: p. 217, it is also useful for gall bladders and kidney problems and for nervous menstrual headaches.

Cancer Chemotherapy, 53:147-151. Smart, C.R. et al. "An Interesting Observation on NDGA and a Patient with Malignant Melanoma."

Author's note: this is a single instance and should not be construed as a treatment to replace current therapy.)

At the University of Utah Medical Center in Salt Lake City, doctors were treating an elderly patient with a malignant melanoma (cancer tumor) that was rapidly growing on his right cheek. He underwent three operations to remove the growth but it kept on coming back. After the third operation without winning the battle and, after the loss of considerable weight and strength, he decided against any more operations.

He went home and began to drink chaparral tea three times a day in 2 to 3 cup allotments. He used 7 to 8 grams of leaves per quart of water to make the tea with. He discontinued all of the medicine prescribed for him and used the tea as his sole source of treatment.

Three months later he returned to the hospital for a check-up. The doctors were amazed to find that the facial lesion was now the size of a dime and the lump in his neck had disappeared.

Six months later he had gained strength and weight and the cancerous lesion was nearly gone.

Chaparral (Croton corymbulosus — Larrea divaricata) contains a substance called nordihydroguaiaretic acid (NDGA) which appears to have anti-cancer potential in tumors as well as leukemia.

The Ethno-Botany of the Maya; Middle America Series, Publication No. 2, Tulane University. Roys, Ralph, L.

The herb, Damiana (Turnera aphrodisiaca) was first used by the Maya Indians of the Yucatan. They used it for all types of lung disorders, dizziness, imbalance, and as an all-purpose body cleaner.

The active ingredients have been isolated and examined because the herb was highly regarded as an aphrodisiac by the ancient Aztecs. At the turn of the century, various products were marketed in the United States to capitalize on its reputation. They were usually 50% alcohol so any so-called effects were probably due to the alcohol and not the herb. Some modern users of damiana have smoked the leaves and said they felt euphoric, relaxed and more imaginative but, according to pharmacologic studies, none of the ingredients could cause those results.

If damiana's reputation as an aphrodisiac is overrated, *Stanford University's Dr. Julian M. Davidson* has the idea that another plant's reputation may be true.

In Cameroon, West Africa, the sacred *Coryanthe johimbe* tree is regarded as a potent aphrodisiac. Its sap, or the synthetic extract called yohimbine hydrochloride, has caused both male and female rats in laboratory tests, to seek out "sexual encounters" at twice the rate of rats that have not been given the herb.

Although it may not be flattering to humans, rats have a sex life that approximates ours. The doctor is now conducting tests to see if the extract will lead to a treatment for human sexual dysfunction.

JNCI 71:855-857, Oct. 1983. Keiko Kuroda. Dept. of Toxicology and Exp. Pathol., Res. Inst. for Chemobiodynamics, Chiba University. Inohana, Chiba 280, Japan.

Fumaric acid is used in the United States as a food additive. It is used as a source of tartness and is generally recognized as safe. It is a component of the herb Shepherd's purse (Capsella bursa-pastoris).

Herbalists have been using this herb as a means of controlling hemorrhages of the stomach, the lungs, and the uterus (Maude Grieve, "A Modern Herbal:" N.Y. 1971; 11:738).

Shepherd's purse also slows the action of the heart, and is capable of elevating low blood pressure ("The Medicinal and Poisonous Plants of Southern and Eastern Africa:" London, 1962; pp. 330-331).

In the Japanese series of experiments which was written up as Kuroda K et al. "Inhibitory Effect of Fumaric Acid on 3-methyl-4 (dimethylamino) Azobenzene-induced Hepatocarcinogenesis in Rats:" the fumaric acid was given to them in their diet and in their water for 51 weeks. At the end of the time, an agent known to cause liver tumors (3-Me-DAB) was given to the rats for 7 weeks.

(Author's note: that's the way animal experimentation is done in Japan, the United States, and in most of the world.)

When the experiment was over, 13.3% of the rats that had been given fumaric acid and the carcinogen had liver cancer *but, 84.6% of the control group which did not have the protection of the fumaric acid had liver cancer!*

According to the research, fumaric acid may inhibit certain types of cancer and further studies should be done.

According to the British Medical Journal *The Lancet*, if fat contributes to colon cancer, a high-fiber diet may help to counteract

fat's deleterious effect by making stools firm and quickening their
transit time through the bowels. The less time fat spends in the bowel
the less chance there is for mutations that cause malignancy.

The journal recommends in descending order: bran, cabbage,
carrots, and apples.

Journal of Food Science, 41:1013-1017, 1976. Konowalchuk,
J. and Speirs, J.L. "Antiviral Activity of Fruit Extracts."

Geraniums are pretty much thought of as common house plants
that you can grow yourself, although their place in herbal medicine as
a digestive and a treatment for heartburn, diarrhea and fever is
mentioned in many herbal tests. Recent studies have demonstrated
their tremendous value in other areas of health. Canadian
microbiologists have learned of the large amount of tannic acid in the
geranium (Geranium masculatum) which represents an effective
antiviral agent against infectious diseases like herpes simplex,
bronchitis, and influenza.

Other plants with this large amount of tannic acid are white
oak bark, bayberry, yellow dock, and witch hazel. The Soviet Trade
Union Journal *Trud* was quoted in the *Calgary Herald* on March 12,
1979 as saying, "Moscow's Institute of Biological Physics has shown
that the acid in unripe gooseberries can prevent the disintegration of
body cells — the very disintegration which causes illness and old age."

Gooseberries (Ribes species) has been called a blood-purifier
and an internal cleanser in herbal lore but this represents a different
view of its herbal ability.

Grapes in the news.

Applied and Environmental Microbiology, 32:757.

Grapes (Vitaceae family; Vitis genera — cultivated) have been
used in folklore as a blood purifier, an antibacterial and as an
antigermicidal. Now, two Canadian microbiologists from Ottawa,
Canada have confirmed that when certain disease viruses were
exposed to fresh and commercial grape juice in the test tube, they
were all killed within a matter of minutes. The viruses affected were

polio, herpes simplex, spinal meningitis, pneumonia, and tuberculosis. They also found that red wines were more effective than white wines.

Montreal Gazette, Wednesday, November 22, 1978.
Scientists have noted that when wounds and sores are bathed with grape juice the infection will immediately stop from spreading further.

National Academy of Sciences, "Herbal Pharmacology in the People's Republic of China;" Washington, D.C., 1975. Ho-Shou-Wu (Polygonum multiflorum)
Most Polygonum species contain leucoanthrocyanidins (LAC) which have been shown to have anti-inflammatory activity, vasodilatory activity, and to decrease blood coagulation.
Since the active ingredients chrysophanol, emodin, and rhapontin occur in garden rhubarb in about the same proportion as in the Chinese plant, it might be wise to resurrect rhubarb pie!

Moscow News, p. 10, June 24, 1979.
The Juniper berry which has been useful in herbal lore as an antiseptic and a diuretic has been made into an ointment for curing deep eye lesions. In addition, a cold liquid extract has been developed as an eye drop. The eye drop, it is claimed, has been successful in relieving glaucoma.
(Author's note: the article did not reveal the method used to manufacture either the ointment or the eye drop.)

Not all herbs are for all of the people all of the time!

Chopra's Indigenous Drugs of India, Calcutta, 1958; pp. 186-187.
Do you love licorice? Does it love you?
Licorice (Glycrrhiza glabra) has been used for congestion, coughs and hoarseness, and as a candy. However, there have been some allergic reactions to it. They include swelling of the ankles, water retention, and an increase in weight.

Patients suffering from heart disease, hypertension, kidney disease, obesity and pregnancy disorders are advised to use caution when offered licorice in any form.

Bestways, June 1979, "Herbal Therapy for the Heart," Potterton, D.

The Lilly of the Valley (Convallaria majalis) contains a substance similar to digitalis. Too much of it taken internally can result in abnormal heartbeat and an upset stomach. It has been used in tincture form in cardiac situations since it increases the muscular action of the heart and the smaller arteries. Since the active ingredient, convallatoxin is rapidly excreted from the body there is little danger of tissue accumulation as there is with digitalis, but, unless you are a doctor, don't eat this plant!

The Lawrence Review of Natural Products, July 1985.

There is a popular folk remedy which uses the dried gum resin obtained from the roots of a shrub called *Ferula assafoetida*. The plant is grown mainly in Iran and Afghanistan and the remedy is as an expectorant, carminative and intestinal spasmodic. Although it is not grown in the United States it is available in drug stores and at ethnic and health food stores.

It is especially popular in the Black community because the Black elderly trust its reputation. The gum dries to a hard, brittle red-brown mass with a putrid, almost nauseating odor and bitter, acrid taste which accounts for its common name — Devil's Dung. If it were not for these drawbacks, it could be a more popular remedy.

Its odor has made it popular in another quarter. A suspension of the substance has been sprayed on fences and shrubs to keep dogs, cats and other wildlife at a distance.

Journal of Dental Research, 63:658. 1984. Rosen, S. et al.

Drinking tea may help to turn white teeth a little browner but may help prevent cavities as well.

Although the data is still preliminary, the study shows that not only may drinkers of the tea have less cavities than non-tea drinkers — but it has two ingredients that fight cancer. One of them is tannin.

Tannins are astringent compounds that may have an affect on the bacteria *Streptococcus mutans* which lives in the mouth and whose metabolic byproducts are largely responsible for the development of cavities.

The other is fluoride. Most teas contain small but potentially significant amounts of this naturally occurring substance, usually in the range of 1 to 2 parts per million. It also comes from the water the tea is brewed in.

The study was done on rats which were fed four types of tea (fluoride content about 1 ppm) for five weeks. Fewer enamel caries were observed in the tea-drinking rats than in a control group that drank nothing but water.

The current study confirms earlier human studies that suggested that tea had a cariostatic effect in children.

(*Caries Research*, 9:312, 1975, Ramsey, A.C. et al.)

(Author's note: this does not mean that you should start your children on tea drinking, even herbal tea, and take them off milk! There are drawbacks to drinking tea. One of them is if you drink tea with your meal you run the risk of the minerals forming insoluble compounds with the tannin and passing out of the body.)

The Lawrence Review of Natural Products, Volume 6, Number 6.

If you've ever travelled by train in the United States you've noticed a tree that lives by the tracks, ignoring all of the pollution and thriving in situations that kill other trees. They have long, slender branches that kids have stripped of leaves and used as whips in imaginary Zorro-games. The tree is the Ginkgo (*Ginkgo biloba*) and is the oldest living tree species. It can be traced back more than 200 million years to the Permian Period. It is the sole survivor of the Ice Age, somehow managing to live in China where it was then cultivated as a sacred tree. The Ginkgo can live to be 1,000 years old, grow to a height of 125 feet, and produce an edible inner seed.

Lately, there have been a number of investigations into the pharmacologic activity that may be present in the leaves. It appears that an aqueous extract of the leaves has some vasodilation action and appears to be effective in treatment of Raynaud's disease although the mechanisms of its action are poorly understood. The extract is generally devoid of adverse effects but contact with the fruit pulp can cause severe poison ivy-like dermatitis. Also, although the seed is edible and sold in Oriental markets, the pulp is toxic if eaten. Luckily, the pulp is foul-smelling and offensive so few people have been tempted to try it or even to pick it up.

The Ginkgo survives where other trees die and continues to do what all trees do, take in carbon dioxide and give off life-sustaining oxygen. What more can you ask of a tree?

University of Georgia, Department of Entymology, Bass, M. and Sheppard, C.

An orange was placed in a cage full of houseflies. Nothing disturbed the flies as they buzzed around and on the fruit carrying on their fly-activity. Then, the orange was removed and the skin was scratched. The orange was then returned to the cage.

Within 15 minutes the flies were acting strangely and in 2 hours, all were dead.

This experiment, and others using different insect pests showed that the oil in orange peels promises to be a natural, powerful all-purpose insecticide.

Natural insecticides are common among plants as they defend themselves against insect predators, the trick is to turn them into something that man can use as well. Tests have shown that orange oil can wipe out fire ants and wasps and kill fleas on a cat, yet does not harm people, animals or the environment. Experiments included placing a damaged orange outside of a cage of houseflies so that the flies had no direct contact with the fruit. The flies still died. When directly exposed to the orange oil, however, they died more quickly. Although Doctor Max Bass, head of the department, said he hadn't tested the orange oil against agricultural pests such as the boll weevil, it looks like we have a potent insecticide against household pests, and one that smells good.

(Author's note: although this is not yet on the market as an insecticide it might pay to scratch an orange and leave it in the fruit bowel. Maybe it will keep flies away and you can write up your own experiment.)

Journal of Nutritional Science, Vitaminol 30:37-46, Jan. Feb. 1984. (Fumitaka Hayase, Department of Agricultural Chemistry, University of Tokyo, Bunkyo-ku, Tokyo.

Antioxidants have made news as nutrition becomes a major weapon against degenerative diseases. Antioxidants help to prevent damage to cells and tissues caused by free radicals that are byproducts of normal metabolism as well as from radioactive sources.

Vitamin E, selenium, vitamin A, vitamin C, etc. are examples of supplemental antioxidants. Now, the sweet potato has joined the ranks of protective nutrition.

An alcohol extract of the sweet potato has been found to have strong antioxidant powers when tested by the researchers. They think it is due ot natural phenolic compounds and amino acids combined in the food.

Not only is the sweet potato good tasting but it is also good for you.

Medical World News, July 23, 1984.

Max Planck Clinical Research Unit for Reproductive Medicine.

A West German researcher told fertility specialists at a conference in Bethesda, Maryland, that healthy grandfathers should be able to become fathers again, since age alone does not seem to impair male fertility. The researcher compared the semen of 22 men aged 60 to 88 who responded to an ad seeking vigorous grandfathers, with that of a group of fathers aged 24 and 37 and found no significant difference. Sperm count, sperm structure, semen pH, semen volume, male sex hormone levels and sperm function were the same in both groups.

Dr. Eberhard Nieschlag, professor of medicine, said, "Impotence and infertility are signs of disease, not age."

(Author's note: I know this has nothing to do with herbs but when I was doing the research and came upon this item, it was too good to pass up.)

"The Sleep That Knits Up The Ravelled Sleeve"

British Medical Journal, November 24, 1984.

Researchers at the Royal Edinburgh Hospital in Scotland have discovered that cell division and protein synthesis reach their maximum values during the hours of sleep and are minimal during wakefulness.

This means that cell rebuilding takes place in the sleep at night. The proper nutrients and a good night's sleep will do more to repair the internal damages suffered during the day than anything else you can do. If this deep, rejuvenating sleep eludes you, then try taking 250 to 500 milligrams of L-Tryptophan at night with or without a glass of warm milk and a cookie. The amino acid is just about as harmless as a glass of milk and far better than prescription sleeping pills since it doesn't appear to interfere with REM sleep.

Bestways, June 1980.

Sea wrack, also called bladderwrack is a seaweed or alga, like kelp, that grows along the shores of the Atlantic and Pacific oceans. Its Latin name is Fucus vesiculosus. It is dark brown, which is typical for algae, with a dull smell and a slightly salty taste.

The active ingredients are iodine, bromide salts and mucous contents. It has been used to treat skin problems and is said to aid in weight reduction, possibly by stimulating the thyroid gland.

If using this for weight reduction, be sure to have a checkup first.

Eastman Dental Center, Rochester, N.Y. October, 1984.

A breakfast of wheat germ, topped with garlic and smothered in rhubarb juice???

Not quite, says Doctor Basil G. Bibby of the dental center. However, rhubarb juice appears to coat the enamel of your teeth with protective mineral compounds, and therefore can slow the decay of enamel as you grow older; wheat germ or bran may act as a buffer against acid (so do peanuts and walnuts); garlic can inhibit the fermentation of sugar into acid (so does sage); and thyme can slow the acidic dissolution of enamel.

Lemons and grapefruits can be bad so rinse your mouth after eating them. Prunes and tomatoes have little effect either way. While an apple at the end of a meal can act as a cleansing agent!

So, vegetarians, rinse, floss, and brush!

Temple University, Dermatology Department.

Your skin has an acid mantle, a protective coating that helps keep it moist and helps keep bacteria at a minimum.

Doctor Ruey J. Yu says that a number of foods can keep that mantle intact and your skin moist. You don't eat them . . . you rub them on your skin.

Apples contain malic acid. Rub a slice of apple on your dry skin.

Sour milk contains lactic acid, another good protecting agent.

Citric acid from oranges and glycolic acid from sugar cane imitate the natural skin acids.

When you sweat you produce lactic acid, one of the reasons that exercise is good for you. The trouble is once you sweat you get into a shower and wash off all that good lactic acid and then you have to use a moisturizer!

About Onions

Department of Medicine and Cardiology, Ravindra Nath Tagore Medical College and Hospital, Udaipur, Rajasthan, India.

The effect of garlic and onion on alimentary hyperlipidemia, induced by feeding butter to 10 healthy subjects has been studied in this research project. The freshly extracted juice of garlic or onion was administered randomly on four different days during the week testing period.

It was determined that garlic and onion have a significant protective action against fat-induced increases in serum cholesterol and plasma fibrinogen.

The conclusion is that the beneficial effects of garlic and onion are due to an essential oil which, chemically, is a combination of sulphur-containing compounds, mainly allyl propyl disulphate and diallyl disulphide.

Onion juice prevented a rise in serum cholesterol after 100 grams of butter was eaten and when garlic juice was added to the meal the serum cholesterol was decreased.

The researchers found that fried onions had some preventive effect on fat-induced increases in serum cholesterol but not as much as raw onion.

It may prove beneficial to use garlic and onion in the diet of persons who appear to be predisposed to atherosclerosis, hyperlipidemia, hypertension, or diabetes.

More About Onions

Dr. Walter Dorsch of the University of Munich, West Germany, has suggested that onion juice can help curb allergic reactions. He injected allergy-producing antibodies into the arms of 12 volunteers. Onion juice was rubbed into one arm and the other arm was left to suffer. The onion-treated arm had significantly less inflammation.

Our Native Americans, the Dakota and Winnebago Indians did almost the same thing. They rubbed wild onion on bee and wasp stings to relieve pain and inflammation.

The active ingredients that have the anti-inflammatory power are still a mystery although Doctor Dorsch suspects they are a member of the isothiocyanate group, so-called mustard oils.

(Author's note: another plus for those countries that cook with a lot of garlic and onions. They have the lowest percent of cardiac conditions in the world.)

Medical University of South Carolina.

Early in the 1970's, Russian animal studies suggested that a substance they called vitamin B-15 could stimulate the body's immune system. They gave this substance, under the name calcium pangamate, to their athletes in the hopes of boosting their performance.

When U.S. doctors examined this substance they found the active ingredient was dimethylglycine (DMG). Traditional doctors said it did not meet the claim of being a vitamin and the Food and Drug Administration agreed with them.

In reality, the substance does not meet the criteria to be called a vitamin since a deficiency of B-15 does not result in any recognizable symptoms and it is not essential to life. But, what about the other claims? It is found in nature and it is a food substance.

Scientists at the Medical University of South Carolina have been investigating DMG and have discovered that it appears to have the ability to boost the immune response and to increase the ability of the tissues to utilize oxygen, therefore releasing more energy. This is what the Russians have been saying for 25 years!

(Author's note: What's in a name? If the substance is useful it makes no difference what we call it. Let's find out if the product can be of help to us. Also, as long as we are investigating Dimethylglycine, lets take a look at Trimethylglycine as well.)

Is There No End
to the Research on Onions?

Scientists at East Texas State University are investigating onion's reputation as an agent to lower blood pressure. Dr's. Moses and Katherine Attrep have identified prostaglandin A-1, a compound known to lower blood pressure, in onion juice. This is the first time a prostaglandin has been discovered in a plant.

Prostaglandins are hormone-like substances that influence many actions and reactions in the human body.

The onion extract successfully lowered blood pressure when injected into laboratory animals but human experiments have not been attempted yet.

Agricultural and Biological Chemistry, 42:1805-6, September 1978. Sakamura, Sadao et al. "Conjugated Serotonins Related to Cathartic Activity in Safflower Seeds."

With the renewed interest in laxatives and regularity and the study of dietary fiber, recent work in Japan has demonstrated that safflower seeds exert a laxative action on the bowels and also stimulate certain glandular secretions within the intestines.

Safflower oil, a polyunsaturated vegetable oil, has been recommended as a substitute for saturated fat in cooking and may have this unexpected benefit as well.

Folk Medicine Vindicated.

Merck Index, p. 558.

A principle constituent of the herb, St. Johnswort, called hypericin, has been clinically employed as an antidepressant in emotionally-disturbed people.

(Author's note: it has been used as a nervine for hundreds of years. Maybe scientists should look into the rest of the "folk tales.")

Journal of Pharmaceutical Sciences, 57:2111-2115. "Hypoglycemic Activity and Chemical Structure of the Salicylates." Fang, V., et al.

The natural pharmacy of the fields and woods, so well understood by our Native Americans, is being investigated for the benefits it can yield to modern living.

The Willow or Pussywillow (Salix alba) contains the glucoside salicin which the body converts into salicylic acid. Modern aspirin has replaced the use of willow bark; however, willow bark may be able to diminish the blood sugar levels in diabetes mellitus, particularly juvenile diabetes, in some cases. This blood glucose lowering or hypoglycemic action of salicin is accomplished by suppressing the release of fatty acids from adipose tissue within the body.

The use of willow bark for headaches and fever was discovered by our Native Americans. The origin is in a fable that may be part truth and part fiction.

The chief of one of the tribes was suffering from a terrible headache and asked the Medicine Man for a potion to relieve it. The Medicine Man responded with a formula that contained as its main ingredient, beaver testicles. The chief drank the potion and his headache was relieved. The Medicine Man became famous and many people asked for the potion.

Father Beaver, the head of the beaver clan was not pleased with the way things were going. The more potion that was being prepared, the less beavers. So, he went to the Medicine Man and proposed a deal. He would show the Medicine Man the tree the beaver chewed on, the tree that provided the medicine that cured the chief, if the Medicine Man would then leave the beaver and his sexual organs intact. The Medicine Man agreed and Father beaver pointed out the willow tree. From that day on, willow bark was used as the medicine of choice for headaches, fevers and colds!

(Author's note: it might not have happened exactly that way but salicin was the basis for the discovery of acetylsalicylic acid which we know as aspirin.)

Journal of Pharmaceutical Science, 58:938-41. "Isolation of the Anti-Inflammatory Principles from Achillea Millefolim." Goldberg, A.S. et al.

Yarrow, a desert herb, has long been used by Native Americans as an anti-arthritic. Now, laboratory analysis has shown that yarrow flowers possess definite anti-inflammatory properties. The oil of the plant does not take part in this action. The property comes mainly from plant proteins and carbohydrates and are the most active in water extracts. Researchers speculate that the proteins and carbohydrates are retained at the site of inflammation for tissue repair. In some cases inflammation was reduced as much as 35% by the administration of yarrow flowers in liquid form.

Vegetarian Times, July/August 1979.

Dr. Chui-Nan Lai, a biologist at M.D. Anderson Hospital and Tumor Institute, has discovered that eating green vegetables will stop the progress of cancer in the colon. Dr. Lai found that extracts of sprouts, particularly from wheat, counteract carcinogens. It was further demonstrated that chlorophyll accounted for most of the extract's anti-cancer effect.

Current tests involve feeding wheat sprouts to cancer-infected mice to determine more exact data on this discovery.

Chinese Journal of Ophthalmology, 1982.

Luffa or loofah is also known as vegetable sponge or dishcloth gourd. It is the fibrous remains of the old mature fruit of *Luffa cylindrica* of the gourd family. Luffa is no stranger to Westerners. We have used it as a body sponge for years to remove dead skin tissue and to stimulate the skin.

Luffa has been used in Chinese medicine since the 10th century. It is said to promote blood circulation, facilitate energy flow in the body, dissipate fever and break up phlegm. It is generally boiled in water and the resulting decoction is taken internally.

But the report in the journal had nothing to do with the conventional uses. It described the use of luffa charcoal in treating three patients with shingles (herpes zoster) in the face and eye region. The luffa was gently heated in a sealed vessel for several hours until it was completely charred. The powdered charcoal was mixed with 50% alcohol to form a paste which was painted directly on the rash.

All three patients were in severe pain and treatment with modern painkilling drugs had not brought relief. Repeated applications with the luffa/alcohol paste completely relieved the pain, absorbed the vesicles, and started the healing process after two days. All patients recovered completely 5 to 7 days after the luffa treatment was started.

Shansi Journal of Medical and Pharmaceutical Health, 1960.

Alfalfa and tooth-bur clover are both called mu xu. Alfalfa (Medicago sativa) because of its purple color is frequently called zi mu xu. Both plants belong to the pea family and have similar active ingredients. Alfalfa is used in the West to treat arthritis and as a source of vitamins, minerals, and plant enzymes.

The Shansi Journal reported the use of mu xu root in the clinical treatment of night blindness. Four out of six patients with night blindness recovered after being treated with daily doses of 1 ounce of a mixture made by cutting the fresh root into small pieces and boiling them in water.

(Author's note: since night blindness is due to an absence of a substance called visual purple which can be caused by a deficiency of vitamin A, zinc, and vitamin B-2, and alfalfa does contain those nutrients, this use makes sense.)

Institute of Nuclear Medicine of the Chinese Academy of Medical Sciences, 1971.

During the past 50 years there have been numerous scientific studies done on the effectiveness of aloe vera gel in treating burns, wounds, chapped and dry skin, leg ulcers and skin conditions. Although these findings have not been conclusive, they do offer substantiation for some of the traditional uses of aloe vera gel.

The remedy published in 1971 uses the fresh aloe leaf to prevent radiation burns.

It calls for blending 30 ml. (about one ounce) of the liquid from the freshly mashed leaf, with 20 grams of gum arabic, plus 0.5 ml. of eucalyptus oil as a preservative and enough castor oil to make 100 ml. (about 3 ounces).

The resulting emulsion is painted on the areas of the skin to be exposed to radiation and allowed to dry.

The Chinese National Pharmaceutical Journal, 1972.

This journal report described the use of chrysanthemum tea in treating high blood pressure and the associated symptoms such as headache, dizziness and insomnia.

A mixture of 1 ounce each of chrysanthemum flowers and honeysuckle was divided into four portions. Boiling water was added to one portion and the mixture was allowed to steep for 10 to 15 minutes. Then the resulting tea was sipped. Each of the other portions was made into tea the same way and sipped at equal intervals. This regimen was repeated for one month. At the end of that time, of 46 patients treated, 35 showed lowering of their pressure and the relief of the other symptoms.

Corn silk, an American herb, is now listed as an official drug in the pharmacopeia of the People's Republic of China and is used as a diuretic and hypotensive in the treatment of edema, nephritis (kidney inflammation), urinary difficulties, jaundice, and hypertension.

Chinese Journal of Internal Medicine, 1960.

Twelve patients with nephrotic syndrome treated by corn silk reported the following: edema (water retention) completely disappeared in nine patients after three months of this simple food treatment. Ten of the patients had severe swelling all over the body before treatment.

The treatment consisted of giving the patients a decoction of 2 ounces of corn silk twice a day along with 1 gram of potassium chloride.

The corn silk came from sweet corn (Zea mays) of the grass family which was cultivated by our Native Americans for centuries. Corn silk consists of the long and slender styles and stigmas of the pistils that stick out from the tip of the corn like a beard.

Corn silk has been used as a diuretic in American folk medicine because the Indians taught the settlers how to use it.

Proceedings of the National Academy of Sciences of the United States and Carcinogenesis, 1982.

In papers presented, American and French researchers reported chlorogenic acid to protect against substances that cause cancer in experimental animals and to prevent the formation of carcinogens such as nitrosamines from nitrites.

The chlorogenic acid the researchers were referring to is found in Honeysuckle flowers, long used as a medicine in China and Japan. Japanese honeysuckle stems, leaves and flowers contain numerous constituents, including luteolin, loganin, secologanin and chlorogenic acid. Chlorogenic acid is believed to be the major active ingredient.

Luteolin is a muscle relaxant, mild diuretic and antibacterial. An extract of the Japanese honeysuckle has been found to have strong antibacterial effects on a wide variety of bacteria.

When Chinese scientists gave an extract of the Japanese honeysuckle to rats on a high cholesterol diet, they found that the rat's blood cholesterol became lower than that of rats not on a high cholesterol diet. They believe that honeysuckle flower extract can retard the absorption of cholesterol from the intestines, resulting in less cholesterol in the blood.

Honeysuckle is not a popular folk medicine in the West but is widely used in traditional Chinese medicine.

The use of Nutmeg (Myristica fragrans) brings to mind Christmas and eggnog in the West. Nutmeg is also used by some fun-seekers for "getting high," because it can produce hallucinations and euphoria, but this practice is very dangerous since the large doses needed to produce the effects can be fatal.

The Journal of Chinese Materia Medica, 1982.

Describes the history and methods of preparing nutmeg, its chemical composition, its therapeutic properties, and problems relating to modern scientific study on nutmeg preparations.

Nutmeg is considered beneficial to the spleen, stomach, and large intestines but it is seldom used alone in Chinese medicine.

Chinese Journal of Surgery, 1961.

Results of the successful use of walnut in treating urinary stones (kidney and bladder stones) appeared to be the most consistent use of walnut. There are four reports. Two in the Chinese Journal of Surgery between 1957 and 1961 and two in regional medical journals.

According to the reports, 4.4 ounces of walnut meat was deep-fried in vegetable oil until crisp. The meat was then mixed with an adequate amount (1 to 2 ounces) of sugar and ground to a milky or pastelike consistency. This milk or paste was eaten by the patient over a period of one to two days. After the patients with kidney and bladder stones took this remedy, their symptoms generally improved in a few days. The stones partially dissolved, turned soft, and then were excreted in the urine.

(Author's note: use of walnut certainly appears to be innocuous and it would not hurt to try, with your doctor's aid, before undergoing more drastic treatment.)

The walnut species used is the *Juglans regia* which is different from the native American species known as *Juglans nigra*. The Chinese walnut is also commonly known as the English walnut.

Better Nutrition, May 1978, 38:54, 56.

Vitamin E and ginseng can help women suffering from "hot flashes" and other menopausal disorders.

National Enquirer, November 9, 1976.

Man confined to a wheelchair due to an accident used a combination of elder flowers, prickly ash bark, yarrow root, burdock root, chives, poplar bark, plus the nutrients zinc, copper, manganese and iron to successfully overcome his condition.

Bestways, July 1978, p. 23.

Some dermatologists believe aloe vera, apricot oil or avocado oil, combined with vitamins A and E will dramatically increase the healing process in cases of burns and the like.

Prevention, July 1978, p. 174.

Letter to the editor: Vitamin C, E, alfalfa, irish moss, yucca, comfrey, chaparral, and burdock helped to clear up a bursitis condition.

Journal of the American Medical Association, 146:760, June 23, 1951.

Studies done by a West German scientist proved that dandelion flowers were very good for correcting night blindness provided that vitamin A and B-2 were added to the treatment. A substance in the dandelions called *helanin* requires the vitamins in order to be activated to help produce visual purple in the eye. The visual purple helps overcome the night blindness.

The Daily Herald, August 1, 1979, Provo, Utah.

Some doctors at John Hopkins Hospital and Medical School in Boston are taking a serious look at the use of medicinal herbs. Dr. T. Bayless, a professor at the medical school is working with Dr. Liang-Yi Cha who believes that certain herbs can work better on a disease than accepted drugs do, and for a cheaper price. Dr. Bayless was particularly impressed with an herbal remedy the Chinese used to remove gallstones without surgery.

Indian Journal of Experimental Biology, 9:376, 1971.

The ancient Ayurvedic medicine of India used myrrh as a treatment for rheumatoid arthritis. Recently two Indian scientists, S. Nitya Anand and N.K. Kapoor, investigated the claims made for this herb. "Pharmacological studies on the crude drug as well as some of its fractions revealed significant anti-inflammatory, anti-rheumatic, and hypocholesteremic activity, providing support for the ancient claims."

Plants of the Bible, Harold N. and Alma L. Moldenke, New York, 1952: p. 159.

Olive oil and fermented olive juice was used in ancient times as a medicinal agent in surgical operations to prevent infections from setting in.

Applied and Environmental Microbiology, 26:777-82, "Anti-microbial Properties of Oleuropein and Products of its Hydrolysis from Green Olives."

During slight fermentation of green olives, a splitting of its enzymes occurred creating a new compound with bitter, phenolic properties. This second compound will inhibit the growth of bacteria and yeasts.

Luke, 10:34.

The Good Samaritan's actions towards the fellow who had been beaten and robbed; he "went to him and bound up his wounds, pouring in [olive] oil and wine . . . "

Planta Medica, 30:39-47, 1976, K. Yamaguchi et al. "The Mechanism of Purgative Action of Geniposide, an Iridoid Glucoside of the Fruit of Gardenia, in Mice."

China has used the fruit of the Gardenia as a laxative for thousands of years. A Japanese pharmacologist investigated the principle active ingredient, *geniposide*. He found that it has a softening action upon hardened fecal material in the bowels thereby substantiating the legendary use of the gardenia.

Cancer   Research,   35:3326-3331;   1975,   Wattenberg, I.W. "Effects of Dietary Constituents on the Metabolism of Chemical Carcinogens."

Alfalfa: Scientists have found that the digestive enzymes in this herb will help neutralize certain forms of stomach cancer.

Texas Dental Journal, January 1966, Bovik, Ellis, G. D.D.S., "Aloe Vera."

A dentist has used liquid aloe vera to bathe sore gums and teeth after recent oral surgery and found it gave great healing relief.

Agricultural and Biological Chemistry, 42:1449-51, July 1978, Setsuo Takeuchi et al. "Benzaldehyde as a Carcinostatic Principle in Figs."

An active ingredient in figs, benzaldehyde, is a very effective carcinostatic agent for reducing certain kinds of tumors found in the neck, throat, and general lymphatic system (particularly the adenoids). How this is done, awaits further scientific clarification in the future.

Indian Journal of Experimental Biology, 16:245-249,   Feb. 1978, V.P. Dixit, et al. "Effects of Malva . . . Flower Extract on the Testicular Function of Dog (Cannis familiaris)."

When the extract of mallow flowers (Malva) was administered to dogs (whose reproductive organs are anatomically similar to that of men), it caused substantial infertility by inhibiting the production of sperm. However, it did not alter any of the other general metabolic activites. Sexual aggression and related impulses remained the same.

It is suggested that oral administration of a liquid extract of mallow flowers for about eight weeks could possibly have the same effect on man as well, thereby limiting his fertility potential while at the same time permitting him the customary response generally experienced with the opposite sex.

U.S. Government Praises
the Health Value of the Papaya.

Department of Agriculture Bulletin No. 77 states:

It is well recognized that the papaya contains peculiar and valuable digestive properties which make it of great value in the diet. These particular digestive properties are largely due to the presence of papain, a very active ferment somewhat similar to pepsin. The papaya also ranks high as a source of vitamins, particularly A and C, vitamins associated respectively with growth and anti-scorbutic effects.

This is all good and well except the department did not say that the largest amount of papain is found in the full-grown but unripe fruit. Papain is obtained by cutting the unripe fruit to let the milky latex or juice ooze out. It soon dries to a powder that is removed and dried in the sun. The dry powder is the basis for many popular meat tenderizers.

The papaya also contains chymopapain which resembles papain in its protein-digesting ability, but is more stable, acid and heat resistant than papain. The U.S. Food and Drug Administration has approved the chymopapain for direct injection (in solution form) into slipped discs.

There have been reports about papain's ability to digest dead tissue without affecting the surrounding live tissue, and this ability has gained it a reputation as a "biological scalpel."

Papaya is healthful and delicious and an aid to digestion.

Need Iron in your diet?
Drink a glass of wine with your meals.

Way back when, an iron nail was stuck into an apple and left there for 24 hours. The acid in the apple dissolved a small amount of iron and when the nail was removed and the apple eaten, the first iron supplement had made its appearance on the nutritional scene.

Later, when mankind got a bit more sophisticated, an iron poker was heated until it glowed, then the poker was thrust into a glass of red wine. The wine was heated (mulled) and, at the same time, some of the mineral dissolved in the wine. So, a second iron supplement joined the ranks.

The next step on wine and iron was a tonic composed of beef, iron and wine which was a popular pick-me-up for iron-poor blood. However, modern science doesn't take wine therapy lightly.

University of the Witwatersrand Medical School, Johannesburg, S.A. Bezwoda, W., Torrance, J., Bothwell, T. et al, "Iron Absorption from Red and White Wines," *Scientific Journal of Haematology*, 1985:34:121-127.

This study compared the iron absorption from a meal containing iron-rich foods when white wine was taken during the meal to the absorption when red wine was imbibed. The white wine won, two to one!

Pediatrics, April 1976.

Doctor Robert B. Elliot, M.D., a physician in New Zealand, has used intravenous infusions of soya oil to bring about some improvement in a small group of children suffering from cystic fibrosis. Soya oil contains linoleic acid which the victims apparently lack. Taking the soya oil by mouth in capsule form or adding it to the diet did not work.

National Arthritis Medical Clinic, Desert Hot Springs, California.

Studies show that saponins from a desert plant were of value in a large percentage of arthritic patients. After daily treatments with tablets made from the yucca extract, 60% of the patients (some of whom had suffered up to 42 years) felt less pain, stiffness and swelling. No allergic reactions were observed, pointing to its safety compared to conventional arthritis medications. The improvement required anywhere from 4 days to 3 months.

Yucca (Yucca baccata, Yucca glauca, Yucca filamentosa,) has been used by our Native Americans for centuries. They used the whole plant. Petals, seeds, fruit, leaves, shoots and roots. All parts are safe and edible. Yucca has been used as a food, a tea, a decoction, an infusion, a poultice, a salve and now, as a tablet. The root can be used for cleansing since it yields a thick lather when it is crushed and soaked in water (it is also known as soaproot) and the Mexican-Americans who have used it claim it prevents baldness.

The Hopi in Arizona use it as a purgative.

The Tewa speaking Pueblo Indians use the fruit to promote easy childbirth.

The Ramah Navaho use a cold infusion of the root for the same purpose.

The Chocktaw make an ointment out of it to heal skin conditions.

The Blackfeet used cut portions of the root to stop bleeding and to allay inflammation. They also used a decoction of the roots to prevent baldness and steamed, grated roots as an anti-rheumatic.

Among Mexican-Americans, yucca is widely used for arthritis. The root is boiled for several hours and the remaining liquid is simmered until it becomes the thickness of a syrup. It is used externally on the sore joint while a tea made from the roots is sipped.

Investigations reveal that the anti-rheumatic and anti-arthritic properties of yucca are due to its saturation with the building blocks of cortisone.

One school of thought is that the yucca saponins improve the body's own production of cortisone by supplying some of the raw materials needed for its manufacture in the adrenal glands.

Singapore Scientist, 1982.

Scientists in India studying the effectiveness of garlic in controlling mosquitoes have reported "impressive" results.

An article in *Singapore Scientist* said that the pungent spice was not only a medical stimulant and an anti-bacterial agent, but also a useful pesticide. Garlic contains two active ingredients that kill mosquitoes on contact.

Warts Soon Gone With Dandelion Juice

Wholistic Health Digest, September 1983.

If you have warts, all you have to do is pick a dandelion flower and squeeze the stem. Touch the wart with a drop of the milk juice and let dry. You may have to do this two or three times, but soon the wart will fall off.

Baylor College of Dentistry, Dallas, Texas

Oral Surgery, 1984:58; 659-666. Thein, D., Hurt, W. "Lysine as a prophylactic agent in the treatment of recurrent herpes simplex labialis."

The effectiveness of the amino acid lysine in the prevention of recurrent lesions of herpes simplex in and around the oral cavity has proved to have mixed, but promising, results. Its use was studied at Baylor College of Dentistry.

The subjects for the experiment had a history of frequent episodes of herpes lesions. They were given a daily dose of either 1,000 mg of lysine or a placebo. After one year of study the group that had received the lysine reported fewer bouts with herpes.

The researchers concluded that lysine might be an effective aid in reducing the frequency of herpes simplex lesions if serum levels of lysine are maintained at optimal concentrations.

Of Men and Plants, Maurice Messeque, Weidenfeld & Nicolson Ltd. Macmillan Publishing Co., Inc. 1973.

One of the greatest herbalists, Messeque, uses garlic, borage, cabbage, corn poppy, watercress, sage and sweet violet flowers in a foot bath to treat bronchial diseases. The garlic is the main active ingredient.

If the idea of soaking your feet in garlic plus other herbs is not too appealing, think about this cure for intestinal worms that was prescribed in ancient Rome.

The patient was instructed to place a number of garlic cloves in his shoe against the skin of the sole of his foot and to walk around that way all day. The oil that was expressed from the garlic was absorbed into the blood stream and circulated to the stomach where it did do the job and kill the worms, but, talk about foot odor!

The Low-Fat Way to Health and Longer Life, Lester M. Morrison, M.D., Prentice-Hall, Inc. 1958.

Dr. Morrison feels that lecithin is the best of all cholesterol-reducing agents tested and that it can help prevent heart and blood vessel disease.

Lecithin is available in capsule, liquid, powder, or granule form in health food stores.

Ohio State University College of Medicine

Dr. R.K. Tompkins speculates that gallstones may be prevented with lecithin. It appears to liquefy the main substance — cholesterol — of which human gallstones are composed.

Journal of Nutrition, 94, 89, 1968.

Everson, G.J. and Sharder, R.E. reported that a lack of manganese can effect glucose tolerance, the ability to remove excess sugar from the blood.

Nutrition Reviews, July, 1968.

In many countries, plant extracts which are good sources of manganese have been used as home remedies in diabetes . . . such as blueberry, onion, brewer's yeast, garlic, seaweed, sunflower seeds and ginseng.

Canadian Medical Association Journal, May 1, 1957.

There have been so many news items about vitamin E and the benefits to the body in the press and on radio and television that we tend to forget that vitamin E was virtually unknown 25 years ago.

However, Drs. Stephen Tolgys and the late, great pioneer of vitamin E therapy, Evan Shute, were publishing the results of the use of this nutrient. In "Alpha-Tocopherol in the Management of Small Areas of Gangrene," they describe vitamin E usage and its ability to save about 50% of patients with gangrene resulting from arteriosclerosis, diabetes, and Buerger's disease, from losing parts of themselves by amputation. They describe, in their 1957 article, how 500 mg. of vitamin E and the use of vitamin E ointment turned black patches of flesh into normal tissue.

Stomach Ulcers Anyone?

Cabbage has been cultivated for over four thousand years and is chock full of nutritive substances. Its value as a food source is not questioned but its use as an aid to heal stomach ulcers was not recognized officially until about the 1950's when Doctor Garnett Cheney, Stanford University Medical School, announced the results of a series of experiments. Cabbage, either eaten raw or juiced, can help heal stomach ulcers.

(Author's note: in my own book, *The Book of Raw Fruit and Vegetable Juices and Drinks*, Keats Publishing, Inc., New Canaan, Conn., I recommend mixing the cabbage juice with carrot juice [one part cabbage to 3 parts carrot] to cut down on the production of gas.)

Science, 1985; 227:934.

We've discovered brain chemicals that influence sex, agression, thought transmission, depression, etc., and now, there appears to be a chemical that influences anxiety!

Marx, J. "Anxiety Peptide Found in Brain."

Alessandro Guidotti, Erminio Costa and co-workers at the National Institute of Mental Health have been working on isolating a peptide which appears to increase anxiety. It is located in the areas of the brain which are important to emotional regulations.

The researchers suggest that the anxiety peptide may act to counter another brain chemical GABA.

What Has Light To Do With Depression?

American Journal of Psychiatry, 1985; 142; 163-170.

Are people more depressed in dim light than in bright light?

Rosenthal, N. et al. "Antidepressant effects of light in seasonal affective disorder."

The authors treated winter depression in 13 patients with typical affective disorder by extending the length of the winter days with bright and dim light in the morning and evening in a balanced-order crossover study. Bright light had a marked anti-depressant effect, whereas the dim light did not.

Several patients were able to maintain the antidepressant response throughout the winter months by continuing the daily light treatments.

(Author's note: we forget how much sun and sunlight influence our well-being. Dr. John Ott has written at great length about light and our pineal gland. There is a new "sunlight supplement" fluorescent light that recreates the full spectrum of the sun and may actually help fight osteoporosis. It's called the Vita-Lite and is available at most stores.)

Sickle-cell Patients Benefit From Vitamin E

American Journal of Clinical Nutrition.

Sickle-cell anemia is a hereditary disease of serious concern for up to 10% of all blacks, and a smaller percentage of people with Mediterranean ancestry. There is no cure for the sickle-cell disease as yet, but recent studies of vitamin E and its effect on sickle-cells may offer hope for an effective way to help reduce the symptoms.

In 1979, Clayton Natta, et al. studied the levels of vitamin E in sickle-cell anemia patients and found that 10 out of 13 patients had less than the standard vitamin E/lipid ratio. Those 10 patients were noticeably deficient in the vitamin.

When they were treated with 450 I.U. of vitamin E from 6 to 35 weeks, the percentage of damaged red blood cells decreased from 24% to 11%.

The conclusion was that vitamin E supplementation could be of benefit to some sickle-cell patients.

St. Thomas' Hospital Medical School, London, England.

Non-drug treatments for PMS (Pre-Menstrual Syndrome), conclude that pyridoxine (vitamin B-6) in doses of 40 to 100 mg is now widely used, especially in less severe cases.

Recent work on the use of the essential fatty acid, gamma-linolenic acid (2-3 g oil of evening primrose per day) has shown encouraging preliminary response.

Other nutritional measures which might reasonably be thought likely to strengthen the wall of small blood vessels are vitamin C, Bioflavonoids, and vitamin E.

British Medical Journal, 1985; 290:417.
Salonen, J. et al. "Risk of cancer in relation to serum concentrations of selenium and vitamin A and E: matched case-control analysis of prospective data."

The independent and joint associations of serum selenium and vitamin A and E concentrations with the risk of death from cancer were studied in 51 case-control pairs — that is, patients with cancer, each paired with a control matched for age, sex, and smoking. The study continued for 4 years.

When the data was analyzed, the conclusion suggested that dietary selenium deficiency is associated with increased risk of fatal cancer, that low vitamin E intake enhances the risk, and that decreased vitamin A intake contributes to the risk of lung cancer among men who smoke and also have a low intake of selenium.

Lancet, Garland, C., et al. "Dietary vitamin D and calcium and risk of colorectal cancer: a 19-year prospective study in men."

The study found that mortality rates from colon cancer in the USA are highest in populations exposed to the least amount of natural sunlight.

Differences in endogenous vitamin D production and calcium absorption could be responsible. To investigate this possibility, the association of dietary vitamin D and calcium with 19-year risk of colorectal cancer was examined in 1,954 men.

The conclusion was that the risk of colorectal cancer was inversely correlated with dietary vitamin D and calcium.

Journal of the American Dietetic Association, 1985; Feb. 1982. Henry, H. et al. "Increasing the intake of calcium conclusively lowered blood pressure: the literature reviewed."

This article cites the evidence in support of an association between dietary calcium and blood pressure. Dietary sources of calcium to provide at least the RDA (recommended daily allowance) are needed. Dairy products are suggested because they supply potassium and magnesium as well as calcium which may assist in the lowering of blood pressure. If a patient cannot tolerate dairy products, oral calcium supplements are advised.

Further clinical investigations are necessary to define the subset of patients who will respond to calcium therapy, but animal experiments and clincal trials support an inverse relationship between calcium and blood pressure.

Preventive Medicine, 1984; 9(2): 7, 16. Bland, J. "Candida albicans: an unsuspected problem."

The prevalence of the fungal infection may be due to the use of antibiotics (without subsequent use of acidophilus to restore the intestinal bacteria), the use of antibiotics in animals, creating long-term, low-level exposure, the use of oral contraceptives which stimulate Candida growth, and nutrient-deficient diets which can alter the intestinal pH and mucosal integrity.

With proliferation, Candida can change from a yeast-like form to a mycelial fungus. The former is non-invasive, whereas the latter produces root-like structures that can penetrate the mucosa resulting in incomplete proteins being introduced into the bloodstream through portals created by the fungi.

The incomplete proteins can influence one's mood, memory, and behavior or cause allergies, acne, headaches and other problems.

Treatment includes yogurt, biotin, olive oil, a high fiber diet, zinc, vitamins A & E and calcium pantothenate.

Archives of Dermalogical Research, 1985; 277:126-130. Cormane, R.H. et al. "Phenylalanine and UVA light for the treatment of vitiligo."

Vitiligo is the loss of pigment in the skin resulting in lighter "patches" on certain body areas. The administration of the amino acid phenylalanine combined with UVA exposure was found to be effective. After four months of treatment, reasonable repigmentation preferentially occurred in the skin area of adipose tissue. After four months of treatment reasonable repigmentation preferentially occurred in the skin area of adipose tissue.

New England Journal of Medicine, 312: 1159-1168. Schneider, E.L., Reid, J.D. "Life Extension."

The effectiveness of interventions claimed to be able to extend life is reviewed. Life expectancy, the average length of life expected by a population, has been increased in laboratory animals by caloric restrictions, exercise, vitamin E, synthetic antioxidants and some drugs.

Life span, the maximum length of life attainable by a member of a species, has also been increased in animals by some of those interventions.

A loss of weight could account for increases in longevity.

Coenzyme Q, interleukin-2, and caloric restrictions may be able to retard or reverse the decline in immune competence that accompanies aging. With the exception of moderate exercise and reasonable caloric restriction in adults, the safety of interventions to produce life extension has not been shown.

Journal of the American Medical Association, 253: 2495-2496, May, 1985. Goldman, D.R. "Hold the Sushi."

Just because fish oil is good for you doesn't mean that raw fish is always prepared correctly. The article warns of infestation with fish tapeworm which may occur after raw fish ingestion; symptoms include nonspecific GI complaints and signs of vitamin B-12 deficiency, or may be absent.

Are "Starch Blockers" about to
Stage a Comeback?

Remember the publicity about the new diet where you could eat all you want of starchy food and you wouldn't digest it so you lost weight while you stuffed yourself?

Gastroenterology, 88: 1895-1902, June 1985. Layer, P. et al. "Partially purified white bean amylase inhibitor reduces starch digestion in vitro and inactivates intraduodenal amylase in humans."

The new nutrient is much stronger and shows much greater power than the crude "starch blockers" that were commercially available before.

The Journal of the American Medical Association, January 1, 1976.

Menopausal or older women frequently complain of a burning tongue that usually involves both sides. When it is due to a lack of stomach acid, doctors prescribe an acid supplement. If the stomach acid is normal in content and strength, a liver supplement plus additional vitamin B-12 and vitamin B-2 (riboflavin) have been known to have good results.

Ob. Gyn. News, December, 1976.

Robert London, M.D., director of obstetrical and gynecological research at Mount Sinai Hospital, Baltimore, Maryland, said that vitamin E can relieve fibrocystitis of the breasts. Out of 12 menstruating women with fibrocystic breast disease, 10 improved in two months on 600 I.U. of vitamin E a day. No cure is claimed, but he said that it seemed to relieve lumps, sores, and tenderness of the breasts, and no harmful side effects have been found.

BEAT OSTEOPOROSIS

FOR LIFE!

Stephen Langer M.D. and James F. Scheer

Know Thy Enemy!

Most magazine and tabloid articles about osteoporosis (weak and porous bones) are dangerously incomplete — as full of holes as the degenerating bones they describe.

The purpose of this chapter is to tell the complete, yet simple story of how to prevent, stop or reverse osteoporosis. And there's more to it than just taking calcium supplements.

Anyone — at any age — can and should protect herself or himself from this dreaded disease which can lead to brittle, painful and honeycombed bones and these telltale symptoms: growing shorter or developing round shoulders, dowager's hump, fractures of ankles, hips or spine — or worse, and even more excruciating, a collapsed spine.

Cause Of The Problem

But before plunging into preventive or corrective measures, let's get into the ABCs of osteoporosis, what it is and what causes it.

In osteoporosis, bones age faster than other parts of the body. We usually think of bones as solid objects that never change, but this is wrong. Like soft body tissues, bones continually lose old cells and develop new ones. This constant tearing down and building up — resorption and formation — affects both the tough outer surface and the spongy inner matter until eventually, withdrawals from the bone bank become greater than deposits. At first though, degeneration is so slow and subtle you don't know it's happening. You can't feel it in your bones.

What Categories Of Persons
Are The Most Likely To Be
Undermined By Osteoporosis?

Mainly women — more than three times as often as men — most frequently, small-boned, short, physically inactive women — or, at the opposite pole — those who exercise so strenuously that their menstrual cycle is interrupted or even turned off.

Other prospects are pre-menopausal women whose ovary has been surgically removed; post-menopausal women; undernourished persons of either sex; drinkers of excessive alcohol or coffee; heavy smokers; those who live and work indoors; the long-time bed-ridden and females and males with many years on the odometer.

Why Is Nature So Seemingly Unfair To Women?

It's nothing personal. On the average, women are more small-boned than men. Their bones are thinner and less dense so, from the start, they have less bone substance to lose before degeneration begins to show.

Several solid studies reveal that women who exercise little physically are decidedly more prone to developing osteoporosis than regular exercisers. This is also true of men, but to a lesser degree.

However, too much exercise of a gruelling nature may be as bad as, or worse than, too little physical activity. According to physiologist Christoper Cann at the University of California in San Francisco, women who habitually work out so hard that they stop menstruating lose bone minerals readily and get an early start on undermining their bone structure. (1)

Even continuous and extreme emotional stress can interrupt the menstrual cycle and trigger destruction of the bone structure, he states. (2)

Estrogen helps to prevent too-early bone demineralization, as many studies indicate. Therefore, says Harry K. Genant, M.D., Professor of Radiology, Medicine and Orthopedics at the University of California in San Francisco, when pre-menopausal women have an ovary removed and stop secreting estrogen, it is as if they are in menopause because their bones start losing substance, durability and strength. (3)

Junky Foods, Junky Bones

Poor nutrition, with the accent on junk foods, creates shortages of many minerals and vitamins — (some of which were never even suspected of having any relation to building and keeping strong bones. A list of these nutrients and the foods richest in them will be given later.) Then, when menopause comes and bones lose their minerals two to three times faster than before, there is little, if any, reserve, which accounts for the many symptoms of osteoporosis, including the 1.2 million fractures of hips, vertebrae, ankles and wrists annually. (4)

Added to deficient nutrition are bone-destructive habits: heavy smoking and heavy alcohol and coffee-drinking.

Why does smoking contribute to osteoporosis? At first, it was hard to penetrate the smoke to get the answer. Then several researchers discovered that menopause arrives earlier in smokers than in non-smokers, and with it comes accelerated bone loss. (5)

Bad Guy Beverages

Drinking large amounts of alcohol daily often displaces the intake of proper foods, eventually causing malnutrition. Further, alcohol attacks and damages certain organs, the liver and kidneys mainly, as well as the brain, and creates greater demands for certain minerals and vitamins. (6)

Coffee-drinking, too, can sabotage bones. As a matter of fact, that great American institution, the Coffee Break, may, in time, lead to bone breaks. Individuals who drink a lot of coffee daily have been found by researchers at Creighton University School of Medicine to be osteoporosis-prone. (7)

Sure enough, one cup a day won't hurt, but two to three cups daily over the years can cause a slow calcium loss. Another aspect of the Creighton study showed that people who drink much coffee usually neglect milk and other dairy products which are rich in calcium.

Enemy Of Bones:
Indoor Living And Immobilization

Even if we take in plenty of calcium, however, we don't necessarily absorb or use it properly without sufficient vitamin D. Several experiments reveal that daily exposure to about 15 minutes of sunlight or skyshine creates enough vitamin D in the skin for this purpose.

On the other hand, individuals who live or work indoors, or who work on the swing or night shift are frequently deficient in vitamin D and in their ability to absorb and use calcium. Round shoulders and widow's hump are common to the northern areas where sunlight is weak — particularly northern Scotland — as they are even in hot and sunny regions of the Middle East where women, for religious reasons, are compelled to keep their heads and bodies covered.

Persons confined to bed for long periods usually develop what is called immobilization osteroporosis, due to lack of exposure to the sun and to little-used muscles and bones. Many studies demonstrate that non-exercising causes flesh to become flabby and bones to demineralize rapidly.

Good News And Bad News

A possible answer to this problem was produced by an experiment at Teijin Institute for Bio-Medical Research in Hino, Japan. (8) Rear limbs of rats were immobilized in a plaster cast. Some of these animals were fed vitamin D for six weeks and then compared with a control group.

Rats on the vitamin D showed a gain of bone weight and more calcium and phosphor, leading the researchers to conclude that the supplementation of vitamin D "diminished the effect of immobilization in the development of osteoporosis without any side effects."

To counteract calcium loss in healthy men kept in bed for reasons of experiment, researchers in the Department of Oral Medicine, School of Dentistry at the University of California in San Francisco, gave these men 10 milligrams of fluoride (recently recognized to strengthen bones in osteoporotic patients) in divided doses each day. However, this measure failed to protect against calcium loss. (9)

Calcium Crisis

When calcium is drawn out of the bones, where does it go? Well-founded scientific observations tell us that just one percent of body calcium circulates in the blood as well as in fluids between cells. However, this amount has to be maintained for wellness — actually, for survival.

So, when the diet is low in calcium or nutrients needed for its absorption and assimilation, the deficiency must be made up by drawing this mineral out of bone structures.

Which structures and in what order?

Fascinating research by Cornell University's Lennart Krook, D.V.M., Ph.D and Leo Lutwak, M.D., Ph.D and associates involved careful examination of jaws and bone structure of periodontal disease patients who had just died from other causes. (10)

In the process, they discovered the priority for calcium withdrawal: first, from the jawbones — as indicated by shrunken jawbones — next from the ribs and vertebrae and, last, from the arm and leg bones.

With shrinkage of the jawbone and tooth sockets, bone draws away from the teeth, loosening them and irritating and inflaming gums often to the point of bleeding.

Early Warning

Degeneration of the jawbone — gum recession or a partly or totally visible tooth socket — is either an early warning that osteoporosis of the skeleton is next in line or that it is already beginning to happen there.

One of the other telltale signs of osteoporosis is translucent skin on the back of the hands, as I observe constantly in my practice. Over and above these signs, self-diagnosis of osteoporosis becomes difficult because by the time the symptoms are obvious, serious degeneration is already underway.

The person becomes shorter. (Overnight, it seemed, one of my patients had to have his trouser legs shortened.) A dowager's hump emerges, or the patient is stricken with arthritis-like pains in bones and joints.

Measurements by means of modern medical instrumentation can offer an early warning of osteoporosis and more time to stop or correct this condition.

X-ray is not the best way of learning for sure that osteoporosis is undermining your bones. Such degeneration really doesn't show clearly until about 30 percent of the bone is lost, as revealed in several experiments.

Bone scanners in many large medical centers can detect early deterioration. So can nuclear magnetic resonance (NMR), which does the job without exposing you to radiation.

Nutrition To Combat Osteoporosis

Osteoporosis needn't even be at work in your mouth, backbone and ribs or ankles or wrists for you to take protective measures.

Additional calcium can be readily obtained from foods such as milk and cheese, and so can the rest of the nutritional ammunition needed to win the battle. However, before creating a special list of foods for this purpose, it would be best to note what vitamin and mineral deficiencies can help bring about osteoporosis and why, starting with the all-important mineral calcium.

Many studies have shown that additional calcium is a good start for defeating osteoporosis — at just about any age. However, the research of Dr. Charles H. Chesnut, Professor of Medicine and Radiology at the University of Washington, reveals that the best way to cure osteoporosis is to prevent it with a super-nutritious diet during the teen years when the skeleton develops its greatest bone mass in terms of size and density. (11)

The amount of calcium taken daily during the teen years really helps to determine the solidity and sturdiness or the porosity and weakness of the bones forty years later.

The Chesnut Regime

Thirty-one 14 year-old girls interviewed by Chesnut were taking from 200 to 1,600 milligrams of calcium daily, from dairy products or in tablet form, with an average of almost 1,000 mg.

Twenty-five percent of the girls were ingesting less than 800 mg daily and were calcium-deficient. One glass of milk provides about 250 mg of calcium. A quart of milk, containing four glasses, offers about 1,000 mg.

A fascinating phenomenon occurred in the girls whose daily intake of calcium in foods and supplements was in the highest range: 1,500 to 1,600 mg. Chesnut found that they absorbed more calcium and retained more in their bones than girls on lower intakes.

Calcium Complications

Dr. Robert P. Heaney of Creighton Medical School in Omaha, a calcium authority, considers the RDA of 800 mg for calcium low in contrast with the 1,500 mg which should be ingested. And a daily intake of 2,500 mg of calcium would help most women without harming them, he says. (12)

For individuals who are milk-intolerant, Heaney recommends alternative calcium-rich foods: sardines, salmon, sesame seeds, soybeans, almonds, brazil nuts, pistachios and sunflower seeds, along with leafy greens.

A much-repeated misconception continues to appear in the popular press about calcium: that a high protein diet — 110 or more grams daily — causes an extravagant calcium loss. This error was rooted in a misread and misunderstood report which appears in the American Journal of Clinical Nutrition, 34, October, 1981. (13)

On a high protein diet, it is true that a greater amount of calcium exits the body in the urine than on a low protein diet, but much more calcium is also absorbed on the high protein diet. In fact, the conclusion of this report is not that a high-protein diet contributes to greater calcium loss, but just the opposite: that it contributes to greater calcium net gain. (14)

Even a diet adequate in calcium can fail to help under two circumstances: if the person eats too many foods with a high phosphorus content and upsets the proper calcium-phosphorus ratio of roughly 2 to 1 or 1-1/2 to 1 in favor of calcium, or if the person does not secrete enough hydrochloric acid to digest foods properly. (This happens often in people as they pass middle age.)

Speaking of tilting the calcium-phosphorus ratio, individuals who eat a lot of eggs, meat, liver and other organ meats and consume many soft drinks — the last-named have a high content of phosphoric acid — lose much of their ingested calcium.

Persons whose ability to secrete stomach acid declines can compensate by taking a digestive enzyme which includes hydrochloric acid in the capsule. (All health food stores carry such products.)

A calcium-rich diet can help most osteoporotic women, even when they are way up in years, as demonstrated by an experiment at Kentucky State University. (15)   Taken aback by the fact that 92 percent of women averaging 70 years of age had slight to marked osteoporosis, the researchers added three slices of cheese and three calcium tablets to the food fare of 20 of these patients for six months.

Using an incredibly accurate measuring technique, quantitative radiography, they checked the density of the women's finger bones prior to and after the experiment. After six months, eleven out of the twenty test subjects showed much greater bone density.   Three retained the same level of bone — an impressive accomplishment in the face of the usual rapid rate increase of bone loss in this critical period — and the six remaining women lost some bone density. However, a total of 70 percent gained bone minerals or held their own.

More Than Calcium

Although calcium is the most spectacular nutrient on the team, the quarterback who gets most of the ink, this mineral needs all the rest of the players to do the job right — vitamins and minerals you might never suspect also have a role: vitamins A, B-6, folic acid, C, D and K, and the minerals magnesium, manganese, boron, copper and zinc. (16)

One of the little-known functions of vitamin A is to help control the process of tearing down old bone cells and forming new ones. (17) When the diet is short-changed on vitamin A, new bone cells are often formed faster than old cells can be evacuated, causing abnormal bone formations which can bring on pain and periodontal problems. (18)

Likewise, vitamin B-6 provides a strong boost towards making good bones happen. A diet low in this vitamin caused rats to develop osteoporosis. And, in a test, more than half of supposedly healthy women volunteers were found deficient in vitamin B-6. (19)

Just how does this nutrient influence bones for better or worse? When well supplied, vitamin B-6 adds strength to connective tissue, the supporting structure of the bones. It also seems to break down and neutralize homocysteine, a harmful substance which appears to contribute to osteoporosis. (20)

Heroics Of Folic Acid

Another of the B vitamins, folic acid, also makes *homocysteine* less poisonous. And methionine, one of the eight essential amino acids, is partly changed in the body to homocysteine. (21)

Individuals with a genetic disorder in which large amounts of homocysteine accumulate are stricken with the worst osteoporosis at an early age, as demonstrated by one study. (22) Before menopause, the body chemicals of women are efficient at translating homocysteine into less harmful substances. After that, they are not. This may account for rapid bone degeneration in post-menopausal women, say some authorities. (23)

When methionine was given to pre-menopausal and post-menopausal women, the latter group showed a greater rise of *homocysteine*. A supplement of folic acid reduced the level of this harmful substance, although none of the subjects tested showed a deficiency of folic acid. (24)

Researchers concluded that there appears to be a greater need for folic acid after menopause. If this need is not filled, poisonous homocysteine levels seem to rise. (25) Studies disclose that 22 percent of persons 65 years of age are folic-acid deficient. Alcohol drinking, smoking and taking of oral contraceptives all contribute to a deficiency of folic acid. (26)

Vitamin C: An Anonymous Contributor

To make cells stick together — in soft tissue and bones as well — the body must produce a glue-like substance called collagen, the most plentiful body protein. A liberal supply of vitamin C is necessary for collagen production.

Without enough of this adhesive, our soft tissue, bone tissue cells and we ourselves tend to come unglued. Vitamin C-deprived guinea pigs showed only a two to three percent tissue content of collagen after 14 days. (27) Animals who continued their usual intake of vitamin C were found to have 14 to 16 percent collagen in their tissue. (28)

Vitamin C also works as a biochemical escort system, making certain that calcium is delivered where needed.

Vitamin D: Calcium Running Mate

The term "Big D," stands for vitamin D, rather than Dallas, because this vitamin enables the small intestine to absorb calcium. So, a deficiency of vitamin D is as serious as too low an intake of calcium.

Too low a blood level of vitamin D is most common in the elderly, particularly elderly women, due to less and less dietary intake, failure to take a vitamin D supplement, a decreased ability to absorb this nutrient and too little exposure to sunlight.

Vitamin D must also be converted to its active form, a process helped along by the minerals magnesium and boron. (29)

The K Ration

One of the best kept secrets in biochemistry is the fact that vitamin K, well-known for its contribution to blood-clotting, is a star performer in assuring strong, solid, healthy bones.

Without it, bones could not be formed, repaired or rebuilt. Vitamin K makes possible the synthesizing of osteocalcin, a protein matrix on which calcium attaches itself to build new bone cells. (30) Osteocalcin is like the chicken wire nailed to the sides of a house so that plaster or stucco can grip the surface. Beyond this function, osteocalcin acts like a magnet to attract ions of calcium. (31)

Because vitamin K is plentiful in vegetables and because friendly intestinal bacteria synthesize it, many nutrition authorities assumed that everybody's blood levels of vitamin K are adequate.

'Tain't so, as is revealed by new and accurate blood testing instrumentation and techniques. Many people avoid eating vegetables or take antibiotics which annihilate the friendly bacteria along with the enemies. Sixteen osteoporosis patients were found to have only 35 percent as much blood serum vitamin K as age-matched controls without osteoporosis. (32)

Both negative and positive animal and human studies show the towering importance of vitamin K. Rats put on a vitamin K-deficient regime lost increased amounts of calcium in their urine. (33)

Healing of rabbits with bone fractures was speeded up when a vitamin K supplement was given, although these animals were already on a diet with a high enough level of this vitamin. (34)

A vitamin K supplement given to human subjects decreased calcium loss in urine by 18 to 50 percent. (35) These research projects reveal that vitamin K may, indeed, be a sleeper nutrient to use as a supplement when dealing with osteoporosis and broken bones.

Mineral Minutemen

When bones are threatened by osteoporosis, the first thing patients think about is calcium. And this is a good first thing to think about.

However, after the calcium is supplied, according to the Chesnut requirement, other mineral minutemen should be called to the rescue: magnesium, manganese, boron, copper and zinc.

Magnesium, a neglected nutrient in the diet of Americans — especially women — contributes to the making of solid, enduring bones by changing vitamin D to an active form and by activating an enzyme that helps create new calcium crystals in the bone.

Concentration of magnesium in body cells and in bones was subnormal in 16 out of 19 women with osteoporosis. Calcium crystal formation in the 16 was defective. (36) This appears to make patients more likely to sustain fractures. Calcium crystals formed in the three women with adequate levels of magnesium were found to be normal.

A Sleeper Mineral

Another unsung hero is manganese — a must for synthesizing connective tissue, structural material in both cartilage and bone, and for assuring that needed minerals will stay put in the bones.

When rats were fed a manganese-deficient diet, their bones were smaller, less mineral-dense and more subject to fracture than those of animals fed enough of this trace mineral. (37)

It was discovered that osteoporotic women had only one-quarter of the manganese blood levels of women who were osteoporosis-free (38)

Bring On The Boron!

Until recent years, even leading biochemists had no idea that the trace mineral boron could be useful anywhere in human nutrition, let alone in bone health and integrity.

One particular experiment rocked them like an earthquake. When three milligrams of boron (obtainable in health food stores) was added to a typical daily diet of post-menopausal women, the amount of calcium which they excreted in urine dropped by 44 percent. (39)

At the same time, their blood serum concentration of the most biologically active form of estrogen rose sharply — to the same level as in the women receiving estrogen therapy.

How does boron work this wonder? Biochemists can only offer an educated guess. When boron joins certain organic chemicals, it appears to make possible the synthesis of the most usable form of estrogen.

It is a well-established fact that estrogen therapy for osteoporosis in post-menopausal women poses certain dangers of cancer. Does this mean that boron presents the same risk? Not really, say authorities.

Oral estrogen must be taken in relatively high doses to clear the gastrointestinal tract and reach the bloodstream in its most effective form. In sharp contrast, the amount of estrogen hormone produced with the help of boron is only about five percent of the oral dose. Therefore, it produces the desired effect with virtually no risk of cancer. (40)

Just as boron helps in the synthesizing of a form of estrogen helpful to bone integrity, it appears to contribute to turning vitamin D into its most useful form. In an experiment with chicks, it was found that a boron deficiency worsened a vitamin D deficiency and made for abnormally formed bones. (41)

A daily intake of only three milligrams of boron appears to bring about dramatic changes in bone formation and strength, according to U.S. Department of Agriculture studies.

The Copper Question

As with boron, just traces of copper are necessary to promote and maintain solid bone structure. A mere two milligrams daily is generally recommended. Surveys indicate that the diet of most people includes about half that much. (42)

Even authorities in nutrition don't know exactly how copper works on body bones, but they are aware of several rat studies which demonstrate that a copper deficiency permits the escape of bone minerals and, therefore, the weakening of bones. (43)

One experiment revealed that copper supplementation blocked the escape of minerals from bones, keeping them solid and strong. (44)

Get In Sync With Zinc!

Noted for its contributions to wound-healing, to a smooth skin, to gland function, including the thymus, the key gland of the immune system, zinc gets little recognition for its part in assuring bone health.

Zinc is needed for vitamin D to be efficient in making calcium take, for bone to form normally and for putting the brakes on too rapid a loss of bone minerals — especially in the jawbone. (45)

Deficiency of zinc could be one of the major causes of osteoporosis, inasmuch as several surveys show that people take in too little zinc. One study disclosed that 68 percent of adults ingest less than the Recommended Daily Allowance (RDA) of zinc. (46) Further, many authorities think the RDA is too low.

Michael Lesser, M.D., in addressing the Senate Select Committee on Nutrition and Human Needs, stated that the soil of 32 states is zinc-deficient and that commercial fertilizers return no zinc to the earth. (47)

Several U.S. Department of Agriculture surveys show the same thing. It is impossible for even a magician to pull a rabbit out of the hat without first having put one inside. Another study revealed that the blood and bones of elderly osteoporosis patients were deficient in zinc. (48)

Added to that, all forms of zinc are not created equal. Some are hard to absorb. Zinc picolinate (available in health food stores) seems to be the form of zinc most readily absorbed, transported and used by the body. (49)

Summary Of Needed Supplements

Over and above calcium, the critically needed supplements for preserving or strengthening bones are: vitamin A, B-6, folic acid, C, D, and K, as well as the minerals magnesium, manganese, boron, copper and zinc.

These supplements and the daily RDA's for them follow:

Vitamin A, 5,000 I.U.'s for men and women. (Various authorities feel that 10,000 I.U.'s are safe.)

Vitamin B-6, 2 to 2.5 mg for adults. (It is difficult to find this vitamin at these low potencies. Generally, vitamin B-6 is present in B-complex capsules or tablets in potencies of 50 mg or 100 mg. Excesses are thrown off.)

Folic acid, 400 to 800 micrograms for adults.

Vitamin C, 50 to 80 mg for adults. (Many biochemists feel that the proper amount could range anywhere from 100 mg to 10,000 mg. At high potencies, this vitamin sometimes has a laxative effect at first.

Vitamin D, 400 I.U.'s. A quart of fortified milk contains about this amount.

Vitamin K. No RDA has been established. However, it is generally agreed by biochemists that 300 micrograms is an adequate daily intake. Above 500 mcg of the synthetic form of vitamin K is considered toxic.

Now for the minerals:

Calcium, 800 mg for adults. Many nutritionists believe that this is low and that 1000 mg to 1600 mg would be a more realistic range.

Magnesium, 350 mg for men and 450 mg for women. Usually, magnesium intake is at a one to two ratio with calcium. So 1000 mg calcium would call for 500 mg of magnesium.

Manganese, five milligrams.

Safe boron intake has been established by the U.S. Department of Agriculture at 3 mg, an amount accepted by most biochemists.

Copper has no established RDA. However, various authorities suggest two to three milligrams.

Zinc, 15 to 25 mg for adults.

Best Food Sources Of These Nutrients

Vitamin A in International Units in 3 3/4 ounce servings:

Cod liver oil	200,000
Sheep liver	45,000
Cow liver	44,000

Calf's liver	22,000
Dandelion greens	14,000
Carrots	11,000
Yams	9,000
Kale	8,900
Parsley and turnip greens	8,500
Collard greens and char	6,500
Watercress	5,000
Red peppers	4,400
Squash	4,000
Egg yolk and cantaloupe	3,400
Persimmons and apricots	2,700
Broccoli	2,500
Pimentos	2,300
Crab	2,200
Swordfish	2,100
Whitefish	2,000
Romaine	1,900
Mangoes	1,800
Papayas	1,700
Pumpkin	1,600
Peaches and cheese	1,300
Eggs	1,200

(Vegetables and fruits contain a vitamin A precursor, beta-carotene, which has to be converted to vitamin A by the liver.)

Vitamin B-6 in milligrams per 3 3/4 ounce units:

Brewer's yeast	4.0
Brown rice	3.6
Whole wheat	2.9
Royal jelly	2.4
Soybeans	2.0
Rye	1.8
Lentils	1.7
Sunflower seeds and Hazelnuts	1.1

Alfalfa	1.0
Salmon	0.98
Wheat germ	0.92
Tuna	0.90
Bran	0.85
Walnuts	0.73
Peas and liver	0.67
Avocados	0.60
Beans	0.57
Cashews, peanuts, turkey, oats, chicken and beef	0.40
Halibut	0.34
Lamb and bananas	0.32

Folic acid in milligrams per 3 3/4 ounce units:

Torula yeast	3.0
Brewer's yeast	2.0
Alfalfa	0.80
Soybeans	0.69
Endive	0.47
Chickpeas	0.41
Oats	0.39
Lentils	0.34
Beans and wheat germ	0.31
Liver	0.29
Split peas	0.23
Whole wheat	0.22
Barley	0.21
Brown rice	0.17
Asparagus	0.12
Green peas	0.11
Sunflower seeds and collard greens	0.10
Spinach	0.080
Hazelnuts and kale	0.070

Peanuts, soy lecithin,
   and walnuts   0.060
Corn   0.059
Brussel sprouts, broccoli,
   brazil nuts, and almonds   0.050

Vitamin C in milligrams per 3 3/4 ounce portions:

Rose hips	3,000
Acerola cherries	1,100
Guavas	240
Black currants	200
Parsley	170
Watercress	80
Chives	70
Strawberries	57
Persimmons	52
Spinac	51
Oranges	50
Cabbage	47
Grapefruit	38
Papaya	37
Elderberries and kumquats	36
Dandelion greens and lemons	35
Cantaloupe	33
Green onions	32
Limes	31
Mangoes	27
Loganberries	24
Tangerines and tomatoes	23
Squash	22
Raspberries, romaine, lettuce, and pineapple	17

Vitamin D in International Units per 3 3/4 ounce portion:

Cod liver oil	20,000
Sardines	500
Salmon	400
Tuna	250
Egg yolk	160
Shrimp	150
Sunflower seeds	92
Liver	50
Eggs	48
Butter	40
Cheeses	30
Cream	15
Human milk	6
Cottage cheese and cow's milk	4
Bee pollen	1.6
Bass	1.0

Vitamin K in milligrams per 3 3/4 ounce units:

Cheddar cheese	22.0
Camembert cheese	16.0
Brussel sprouts	1.5
Soy lecithin	1.2
Alfalfa	0.52
Oats	0.49
Spinach	0.33
Soybeans	0.30
Cauliflower	0.28
Cabbage	0.25
Broccoli	0.20
Liver	0.10
Potatoes	0.08
Bran	0.069
Watercress	0.060
Peas	0.044

Beef	0.035
Wheat germ	0.033
Tomatoes	0.027
Honey	0.025
Strawberries	0.013
Eggs	0.012
Carrots, corn and asparagus	0.010

Calcium in milligrams per 3 3/4 ounce servings:

Sesame seeds	1,200
Kelp	1,100
Cheeses	700
Sea salt	670
Brewer's yeast	420
Sardines and carob	350
Caviar	280
Soybeans and almonds	230
Torula yeast	220
Parsley	200
Brazil nuts	190
Watercress, salmon and chickpeas	150
Egg yolk, beans, pistachios, lentils and kale	130
Sunflower seeds and cow's milk	120
Buckwheat	110
Maple syrup, cream and chard	100
Walnuts	99
Endive	81
Pecans	73
Wheat germ	72
Peas	70
Peanuts	69
Eggs	54
Oats	53

Magnesium in milligrams per 3 3/4 ounce units:

Kelp	740
Blackstrap molasses	410
Sunflower seeds	350
Wheat germ	320
Almonds	270
Soybeans	240
Brazil nuts, bone meal	170
Pistachios and soy lecithin	160
Hazelnuts	150
Pecans and oats	140
Walnuts	130
Brown rice	120
Chard	65
Spinach	57
Barley	55
Coconut	44
Salmon	40
Corn	38
Avocados	37
Bananas	31
Cheeses	30
Tuna	29
Potatoes and cashews	27
Turkey	25

Manganese in milligrams per 3 3/4 ounce units:

Seaweeds	120.0
Tea leaves	28.0
Cloves	26.0
Ginger	8.7
Buckwheat	5.1
Oats	4.9
Hazelnuts	4.2
Chestnuts	3.7

Wheat	3.6
Pecans	3.5
Barley	3.2
Brazil nuts	2.8
Sunflower seeds	2.5
Watercress, peas, beans	2.0
Almonds	1.9
Turnip greens, walnuts	1.8
Brown rice	1.7
Peanuts	1.5
Honey	1.4
Coconut	1.4
Pineapple	1.1
Parsley	0.94
Spinach	0.82
Grapefruit and lettuce	0.80
Bananas	0.64
Carrots	0.60
Brewer's yeast	0.53
Yams	0.52
Kale	0.50

An in-depth study has not been completed on boron-containing foods. However, here are some of the foods richest in boron without the number of milligrams given per 3 3/4 ounce servings: apples, legumes, nuts, pears, leafy vegetables, soy meal, prunes, raisins, almonds, peanuts, hazelnuts, dates and honey.

Copper in milligrams per 3 3/4 ounce servings are:

Liver	3.7
Wheat germ	2.9
Thyme	2.4
Blackstrap molasses	2.2
Black pepper	2.1
Honey	1.7
Hazelnuts	1.4

Brazil nuts	1.1
Walnuts	0.90
Kelp and salmon	0.80
Cashews	0.76
Oats	0.74
Lentils	0.71
Barley	0.70
Almonds	0.68
Bananas	0.51
Tuna	0.50
Avocado and coconut	0.39
Brown rice	0.36
Bee pollen	0.32
Eggplant and kale	0.30
Chicken	0.28

Zinc in milligrams per 3 3/4 ounce servings:

Herring	110.0
Wheat germ	14.0
Sesame seeds	10.0
Torula yeast	9.9
Blackstrap molasses	8.3
Maple syrup	7.5
Liver	7.0
Soybeans	6.7
Sunflower seeds	6.6
Egg yolk	5.5
Lamb	5.4
Chicken	4.8
Brewer's yeast	3.9
Oats	3.7
Rye	3.4
Whole wheat	3.2
Corn	3.1
Coconut and beef	3.0
Beets, turkey and walnuts	2.8

Barley	2.7
Beans and avocados	2.4
Peas	2.3
Bleu cheese	2.2
Eggs	2.1
Buckwheat	2.0
Mangoes	1.9
Millet, brown rice and almonds	1.6
Salmon	1.4

The Estrogen Dilemma

After menopause, estrogen production sharply declines and, consequently, bone loss increases. Borje E. C. Nordin, of the Royal Adelaide Hospital in Adelaide, Australia, discovered much lower estrogen levels in post-menopausal women with osteoporosis than in healthy post-menopausal women. (50)

There are still many mysteries as to how low levels of estrogen speed up bone demineralization. However, many studies demonstrate convincingly that estrogen therapy does prevent excess bone loss in healthy post-menopausal women.

Dr. Robert Lindsay, an osteoporosis authority at Helen Hayes Hospital in West Haverstraw, New York, conducted an experiment which revealed that estrogen replacement can prevent spinal fractures — a medical nightmare — in healthy post-menopausal women. (51)

Yet many medical doctors who favor estrogen therapy for preventing or slowing osteoporosis do not routinely prescribe it for this purpose because it poses a risk of uterine cancer. Conscientious and responsible doctors make patients aware of the risk factor.

Consequences Of Ovarian Surgery

Harry K. Genant, M.D., Professor of Radiology, Medicine and Orthopedics at the University of California at San Francisco, made a thorough survey of the critical problem of rapid bone loss after menopause. Bone loss in the spine of women whose ovaries had been surgically removed was frighteningly rapid, 7 to 9 percent annually on average. (52) Some women lost as much as 15 to 20 percent.

Genant's research with the spine was the first of its kind and also revealed that women who go through menopause naturally lose bone minerals more slowly than women with surgically-induced menopause (five percent annually, still a threatening rate). (53)

The cancer threat is real because Dr. Genant's study disclosed that only a high-dosage of estrogen, 0.6 mg, could manage osteoporosis. Five out of six patients lost no bone on the 0.6 mg dosage and some even recovered a small amount of bone minerals. (54)

Favorable results scored by boron in post-menopausal women give hope that this trace mineral might eliminate or at least minimize estrogen therapy and its accompanying danger.

Another alternative to estrogen therapy with its possible hazard is taking the supplement calcium lactate, or calcium carbonate if the person cannot tolerate milk or other dairy products, states an article in the conservative New England Journal of Medicine. (55)

Exercise: Another Dimension In
Bone-Building

Several studies indicate that how you exercise is as important to preventing, neutralizing or reversing osteoporosis as how you eat.

All right. What are the exercise best bets?

Jogging, running, or tennis, state Peter Jacobson and associates at the University of North Carolina in Chapel Hill, who have done much experimentation in this field. (56)

Now, hear this! Some osteoporosis has gone so far that exercise could cause bone collapse, so it's best to have your doctor check you carefully before okaying an exercise program.

Jacobson says that weight-bearing exercise can often counter bone loss after menopause.(57) He compared post-menopausal women who played tennis three times a week with age-matched non-exercising women. The tennis players had much more bone mass than the sedentary test subjects, accenting the fact that exercise can slow or prevent bone loss.

Best Bone-Building Exercises

Aerobic dancing not only melts off the surplus suet, it is also a phenomenal activity for coping with osteoporosis, as discovered by R. Bruce Martin, M.D., Director of Orthopedic Research at West Virginia Medical Center. (58)

Martin and co-workers tested several exercises on middle-aged women, the prime test subjects because bone demineralizes most rapidly in the ten years following menopause.

One group did aerobic dancing. A second group walked two miles a day four times each week. The third group's only exercise was avoiding exercise.

"Before" and "After" tests made a striking impression on the researchers and the patients, too. After six months, the non-exercisers had lost 1.5 percent of calcium and other major minerals in an arm bone.

The walkers, too, lost some bone minerals, but not quite as much. However, the aerobic dancers lost none of the key minerals in the arm bone, supposedly because they exercised both arms and legs in dancing. The dancers and walkers showed a marked gain: greater width of the arm bone.

Doing The Impossible:
Reversing Osteoporosis

It is possible to beat osteoporosis by exercise and Everett L. Smith, Ph.D., an authority on the biology of aging at the University of Wisconsin in Madison, has the statistics to prove this point. (59) He found that the throwing arm of young baseball pitchers and the arm wielding the tennis racket have much more bone mineral mass than the other arm.

Dr. Smith also studied older tennis players — those averaging 64 years of age — and found the identical condition in their dominant arm.

Then he studied thirty-eight women who were an average of eighty-four years old, dividing them into two groups: eighteen non-exercisers and twelve who performed physical activity a half hour each week for three years. Each exerciser sat on a chair and performed 103 different movements, motions calculated to utilize most of the body bones.

Three years later, the non-exercisers showed a loss of 3.29 percent of their bone minerals. In sharp contrast, the exercisers revealed a gain of 2.29 percent of the bone mineral content. The Smith experiment shows it's never too late.

Summing Up

If diet on its own can stop or even reverse osteoporosis and exercise can do the same, why not combine an optimized diet with an optimized exercise program?

This two-front war on osteoporosis can defeat an enemy which never quits, silently working to break your bones and you.

The previous pages map out a campaign strategy that exists in no other publication. All you have to do is take command and follow the strategy.

Victory over osteoporosis is yours. Can't you feel it in your bones?

References

1. "Bone Loss Linked to Early Menstruation Halt," *Register* (Orange County, CA), February 3, 1984): Section B, 10.
2. Ibid.
3. "Bone Disease Found to Strike the Young, Too." Associated Press Release (September 14, 1983).
4. "Nutrients and Bone Health," Wright/Gaby Nutrition Institute, August, 1988, 1.
5. *Practical Encyclopedia of Natural Healing* (Emmaus, PA.: Rodale Press, Inc., 1982): 70.
6. Ibid.
7. Ibid.
8. Izawa, I., et al, *Calcification Tissue International*, 36 (1981): 623-30.
9. Meshawari, U.R., et al, *American Journal of Clinical Nutrition*, 36 (2) (1982): 211-18.
10. *Practical Encyclopedia*: 493-494.
11. *Los Angeles Times*, June 25, 1986, Part II, 1.
12. "Bone Disease May Cripple Older Women," *Los Angeles Times*, (August 19, 1983).
13. *American Journal of Clinical Nutrition*, 34: (October, 1981): 2178-2186.
14. Ibid.
15. Ibid.
16. "Nutrients and Bone Health," Wright-Gaby Nutrition Institute, August, 1988, 1.
17. *The Complete Book of Vitamins*, (Emmaus, PA.: Rodale Press, Inc., 1977): 136.
18. *The Complete Guide to Health and Nutrition*, Gary Null (New York, N.Y.: Dell Publishing Co., Inc., 1984): 243-244.
19. "Nutrients and Bone Health," Wright/Gaby Nutrition Institute, August 1988, 3.
20. Ibid., 2.
21. Ibid.
22. Ibid.

23. Ibid.

24. Ibid.

25. Ibid.

26. Ibid.

27. Long, Ruth Yale, *Home Study Course in the New Nutrition*, (New Canaan, CT.: 1989): Lesson 9, 10.

28. Ibid.

29. "Nutrients and Bone Health," Wright/Gaby Nutrition Institute, August, 1988, 2-3.

30. Gallop, P.M., et al, Carboxylated Calcium-Binding Proteins and Vitamin K, *New England Journal of Medicine*, 1980; 302: 1460-1466.

31. Ibid.

32. Hart, J.P., et al, Electrochemical Detection of Depressed Circulating Levels of Vitamin K in Osteoporosis, *Journal of Clinical Endocrinology and Metabolism*, 1985; 60: 1268-1269.

33. Robert, D., et al, Hypercalciuria During Experimental Vitamin K Deficiency in the Rat, *Calcification Tissue International*, 1986; 37: 143-147.

34. Ibid.

35. Ibid.

36. Cohen, L., Kitzes, R., Infrared Spectroscopy and Magnesium Content of Bone Material in Osteoporotic Women, *Israeli Journal of Medical Science*, 1981; 17: 1123-1125.

37. Amdur, M.O., et al, The Need for Manganese in Bone Development by the Rat, *Proceeding of the Society of Experimental Biological Medicine*, 1945; 59: 254-255.

38. Raloff, Janet, Reasons for Boning Up on Manganese, *Science News*, 1986 (Sept. 27): 199.

39. "Nutrients and Bone Health," Wright/Gaby Nutrition Institute,August, 1988, 3.

40. Ibid.

41. Ibid.

42. Hyams, D.E., Ross, E.J., "Scurvy Megaloblastic Anaemia and Osteoporosis," *British Journal of Clinical Practice*, 1963; 17: 332-340.

43. "Nutrients and Bone Health," Wright/Gaby Nutrition Institute, August, 1988, 3.
44. Ibid.
45. Ibid.
46. Ibid.
47. Langer, Stephen and Scheer, James F., "How to Win at Weight Loss," (Rochester, VT.: Thorsons Publishers, Inc. 1987): 66.
48. Atik, O.S., "Zinc and Senile Osteoporosis," *Journal of the American Geriatric Society*, 1983; 31: 790-791.
49. "Nutrients and Bone Health," Wright/Gaby Nutrition Institute, August, 1988, 3.
50. "Boning Up on Osteoporosis," *Science News*, Vol. 124 (July 27, 1983): 141.
51. Ibid.
52. "Treating Post-Menopausal Bone Loss," *Los Angeles Times*, (February 27, 1983), Part VII, 20-21.
53. Ibid.
54. Ibid.
55. *Practical Encyclopedia*, 75.
56. "Boning Up on Osteoporosis," *Science News*, Vol. 124 (July 27, 1983): 140.
57. Ibid.
58. "Bone Disease May Cripple Older Women," *Los Angeles Times*, (August 19, 1983).
59. *Practical Encyclopedia*, 172.

DIETAL WEAPONS
AGAINST
MENOPAUSE

Dr. William H. Lee

DIETAL WEAPONS AGAINST MENOPAUSE

Normal Symptoms of Menopause and Why

Human females get an extra added bonus from nature. Unlike other species, they live beyond the time of their fertility and child-bearing. Improved environmental conditions and a better understanding of what really goes on inside their bodies have resulted in a considerable lengthening of this span.

A thousand years ago, the average age of death for a women was approximately 30 years.

When Elizabeth I was queen, the average demise was lengthened to age 40. And, it was not until the 20th century that death approximated the appearance of menopause at about age 50.

Now, barring unforeseen circumstances, it is not uncommon to find that women can enjoy 25 years or more of a happy, productive life after menopause.

The entrance of more women into the medical profession and a more enlightened look at it has altered the previous male-dominated viewpoint as "merely a state of mind," to its present state as a hormonal deficiency disorder.

The new attitude is a far cry from that of just a few years ago when the subject was rarely discussed — being concerned, after all, with reproduction and feminine organs. However, even though the attitude has changed, a lot of the ignorance and misinformation still persists.

That women commonly experience problems with menopause is well known. Television has even popularized hot flashes, weaving them in and out of such programs as "Golden Girls." One of the first studies of menopause occurred in the early thirties in England. The *British Medical Women's Federation Report* reported that their study revealed that only a small number of women, about 15 percent, went through menopause without having distressing symptoms. The resulting effect of the discontinuation of the reproductive cycle can range from mild to devastating . . . but nowadays, controllable!

Symptoms & Medical Problems

* Hot flashes, sweating, chronic itch
* Rheumatic-like pains
* Loss of vaginal lubrication and elasticity (can interfere with normal intercourse)
* Sleep disturbances
* Weight gain
* Hair and skin changes (not for the better)
* Change in breast size
* Increased incidence of bladder symptoms such as frequency and often a burning feeling when urinating
* Psychological problems, including:
  depression
  loss of self-esteem
  anxiety
  poor memory
  loss of emotional control
  inability to cope with daily problems
  reduced desire for sexual contact

This formidable list of symptoms, which used to be "only in their heads," can be considered to be the immediate problems of the menopause, but there are also delayed symptoms which can be more serious.

Osteoporosis, which is characterized by a significant thinning of the bones due to a drop in estrogen levels which causes a loss of calcium and other bone chemicals, may lead to fractures of the hip, spine or wrist bones. According to a Mayo Clinic study more than 150,000 hip fractures are directly tied to osteoporosis every year.

The bone thinning of osteoporosis and/or "dowager's hump," can be countered with dietary calcium. Calcium can be obtained from food, but the quantities needed are usually greater than can be obtained from a normal diet. Therefore, the use of calcium supplements are strongly advised. 1000 milligrams to 1,500 milligrams of elemental calcium appear to be desirable. This would be a daily dose. Consider taking a multiple mineral supplement while you're shopping for minerals. Here's a dynamite combination of nutrients that you can easily whip up at home that should do the job:

Calcium Carbonate and Calcium Lactate—to add up to
    1,000 to 1,500 milligrams
Silica—100 milligrams
Zinc—10 to 20 milligrams
Boron—3 milligrams

Other problems may include diseases of circulation (stroke, heart attack, atherosclerosis). It appears that nature protects women during the child-bearing years and makes them less prone to these diseases than men. However, after menopause, women catch up to men as far as these risks are concerned.

Why Does This Happen?

Ovaries (there are two of them) have a lifespan limited to their activity. At the time of puberty each ovary contains about 200,000 eggs and every month some of these eggs mature and one of them will turn into a small gland known as the corpus luteum. The corpus luteum manufactures the two female hormones known as progesterone and estrogen.

Once the ovaries have exhausted their supply of eggs there is no way they can be brought back to an active position. That's a fact that must be accepted. At menopause, not one egg remains in a living condition. Therefore, it follows that the ovary can no longer manufacture progesteron and estrogen. It is the loss of these female hormones that is the cause of all of the troubles.

In a way, menopause is the wrong term to use for the period of time that follows the end of fertility. The menopause is only the stopping of menstruation. The true term is the climacteric, a period of time during which a new endocrine equilibrium is established in which the ovaries have no part. The climacteric really starts months or even years before the final cessation of the ovarian function and the hormone output is slowly reduced, not cut off all at once. This may be the reason some women go through menopause and the climacteric with hardly a twinge.

Although the ovaries slowly or suddenly stop churning out hormones, the body is not put together without a backup system. The ovaries cease egg production. They have been working for years under the guidance of the pituitary gland seated in the base of the brain. The pituitary has been sending chemical messengers (FSH and LH) since puberty as stimulants causing the secretion of the hormones. At the menopause, when the ovaries can no longer respond to the urging, the pituitary responds by increasing the messengers to try to re-awaken the ovarian capacity. No luck! Once it's over it's over . . . but the pituitary can't accept the idea and keeps sending out FSH and LH. In fact, one of the tests to determine menopause is to find large amounts of FSH and LH in the blood.

It is thought that one of the first symptoms of menopause that a woman notices is probably hot flashes. These produce sensations of intense heat followed by clamminess and are usually accompanied by a visible flushing, heavy perspiration, palpitations and sometimes nausea and anxiety. They may be set off by the unregulated release of LH (lutenizing hormone).

NOTE: Some women have found that it is opportune to dress in layers so they may add or shed clothing as their body temperature fluctuates.

If hot flashes become a nightly event they can interfere with normal sleep patterns. The person can become drenched in sweat and have to get up to change nightclothes and sheets. This interruption of sleep may lead to fatigue, irritability and erratic behavior duing the following day. Acceptance of this nighttime hot flash, instead of annoyance, will be a great help to restoring a restful night's sleep.

The body's backup system includes the adrenals and other glands which begin to step up their activity to compensate for the loss of ovarian activity. The adrenals, being the glands of stress, and already over-burdened because of the standard American diet (SAD), excess sugar and ecological and environmental insults, need a diet which support their activity. Whole grains, steamed vegetables, fresh fruit, fish and fowl, brown rice and no cigarettes, alcohol, refined flour and table sugar. Also herbal teas and herbal capsules, nutritional supplements to balance the body's new needs, exercise (including Kegal exercises, more about that later on) and lifestyle changes will make you feel a lot better and get you through the worst of it.

Remember: as your estrogen level declines you metabolize fat at a more sluggish rate so it's easier to gain weight. You have to combat middle-age spread by controlling the number of calories you take in.

Many problems are preventable — or even reversible!

Estrogen Therapy

It's yours if you want it!

If you consider menopause to be a disease then treat it as a disease. Go to your doctor and have him prescribe estrogen or related drugs. Estrogen replacement therapy (ERT) uses drugs like Premarin (conjugated estrogens), estropipate, ethinyl estradiol, to treat moderate to severe symptoms and, to be honest, does help in many cases. However, the possible side effects can be frightening and should be understood before beginning estrogen therapy. Have your doctor explain it all to you in full!

If you consider menopause to be a natural process, then consider using natural methods. We'll go into a lot of different products and substances as you go further into this chapter, but here's some of the things you'll read about:

Ginseng

Cools down hot flashes immediately and amazingly. Why? Because Ginseng contains a safe natural-food variant of estrogen.

Vitamin E Plus
the Mineral Selenium

By smoothing out hormone fluctuations, it helps relieve all menopausal and post-menopausal symptoms. Use 400 I.U. of vitamin E and 200 micrograms of selenium.

L-Tryptophan

An amino acid that helps evaporate "over-fifty" depression and sleep problems. Can be taken in 2 tablet doses at night for sleep and one tablet during the day for anxiety.

The B-Complex Vitamins

They help the adverse emotional and physical effects of stress associated with menopause. You can take a B-Complex 50 tablet twice or three times a day during difficult times. The B-Complex and vitamin C are soluble in water and are easily lost from the body.

Herbals

Chamomile tea is a good calming herbal. It comes alone or in combination. Passiflora tea is also calming. A capsule of Valerian is as effective as valium but not habit forming. (More about herbs later on.)

Bones

Need Calcium and Magnesium plus other minerals to avoid osteoporosis.

Calcium absorption can be interfered with by the tannic acid in tea, the oxalic acid found in rhubarb and spinach, by phytic acid found in grains, by drugs such as aspirin — antibiotics — diuretics — anti-convulsant medicines — aluminum-containing antacids — and excessive coffee drinking.

A high protein diet can also cause calcium loss so balance your intake of protein with adequate grains and vegetables. Avoid excessive consumption of soft drinks with their phosphoric acid content.

Nutritionists consider menopause to be a perfectly natural process which, if prepared for with the proper diet and use of supplements, can be relatively calm and comfortable for the healthy, well-nourished woman. It is true that the "shifting of gears" requires a slightly different approach to life. After all, the freedom from monthly discomforts and the freedom from possible pregnancy has to add some zest to your love life as long as the sexual organs are capable of normal function. They will be, as long as adequate vitamin A and E plus the B-Complex are available to the body. Almost at once, the adrenals take over with the production of a hormone that is similar to estrogen.

Doctors are aware of this but they don't appear to have the time to tell their patients, at least in most cases. If they would take the time to help women build up their own glands so that women could rely on their bodies when the transition time comes, the menopause would be smoothed over and problems would be non-existant. But, most medical men resort to estrogen therapy which can bring on its own set of problems. Some women go on estrogen for years and then, when they finally decide to stop, find themselves experiencing the very same symptoms for which they were given estrogen in the first place.

The adrenals are the anti-stress headquarters for the body and women during menopause are certainly stressed. Therefore, the adrenals, as the only internal source of hormones, must be supported and nourished. The adrenals need loads of pantothenic acid (one of the B-Complex vitamins). Even if you are taking a B-Complex 50 tablet three times a day, you may need an additional 50 to 100 milligrams of pantothenic acid for a few months, or at least until the worst symptoms have gone away.

Besides pantothenic acid, vitamin C is important to the health of the adrenal glands. Some experiments done on guinea pigs who do not produce their own vitamin C (we can't either) show that the need for vitamin C increases 75 fold during and after menopause. This translates roughly into about 5,000 milligrams a day for humans.

Protein is needed by the adrenals. It is reasonable, since hormones are manufactured from protein. Fish, chicken, rice and beans, nuts and seeds are good protein sources. Potassium is also important. The potassium/sodium relationship has been explained. Try bananas, blackstrap molasses, beans, parsley, wheat germ, sesame seeds and avocados.

Dietary and nutritional supplementation directed to helping the adrenals do their job and improving their function is one of the most helpful natural, non-drug approaches to menopause.

Saul Gusberg, M.D., a gynecologist at Mount Sinai Hospital in New York City supports the concept that thre is no reason for estrogen replacement therapy, especially when the severity of the symptoms can be directly traced to nutritional deficiencies. The reduction of estrogen does deplete the woman's supply of vitamin B-2 (riboflavin), vitamin B-6 (pyridoxine), vitamin B-12 (cobalamin), folic acid, vitamin C (ascorbic acid), vitamin E (tocopherol) and the minerals calcium, magnesium, zinc, chromium, potassium and phosphorus, among other needed nutrients.

Nutritional replacement therapy designed to use greater-than-recommended amounts of vitamins and minerals will help reduce the physical and mental symptoms. Simply replacing these lost minerals will dramatically reduce the chances of "dowager's hump," the spinal compression resulting from bone loss and loss of height, as will replacing vitamin B-12, either by injection, with tablets, or by eating foods such as liver, clams, kidneys, oysters, sardines, eggs, trout, brains, salmon, tuna, sweetbreads, Edam cheese, Brie cheese, Gruyere cheese, haddock, flounder, scallops, halibut, perch, or swordfish.

Nutritional replacement therapy can begin before menopause if the woman will eliminate sugar, refined flour and "junk food" from the diet while adding the beneficial foods and using nutritional supplements to shore up the body's reserves before they are needed. Among the best resources are vitamin E, ginseng, and Gamma linolenic acid (GLA)

We already know that ginseng curbs hot flashes and energy loss. We know that the body is in a state of stress. Since ginseng is able to naturally stimulate the body to produce a balancing supply of hormones it helps to normalize the situation. One or two 650 milligram capsules as a tea or swallowed daily should help. Like many natural remedies, it takes a while to see results. If there are no side effects, three to six weeks of nutritional therapy for satisfactory progress is the usual time span.

Vitamin E is an excellent natural alternative to estrogren therapy according to Warren E. Levin, M.D. medical director of the World Health Medical Group in New York City. He says a nutritional approach takes longer than estrogen therapy (about six months) but it can do a better job than anything else.

Gamma-linolenic acid is a direct precursor for the body's production of prostaglandins (hormone-like substances) which direct the second-by-second activities of the system. When taken with vitamin E, it supports the body's efforts to do away with painful breast lumps. One or two capsules two or three times a day is the usual regimen.

Estrogen Promoting Foods & Herbs
And What Else Foods Can Do

Some foods we eat have either estrogenic or progesteronic activity. Continually eating the wrong foods can wreak havoc during the menopause.

Some foods contain plant steroids and flavonoids that are relatively inactive until they are acted on by intestinal bacteria. Then they are transformed into functioning sexual hormones. These hormones can then be absorbed by the body.

Other natural food constituents can act against estrogenic action.

On the whole, estrogen promoting foods and herbs should be added to the diet for symptoms of menopause.

Estrogen Promoting Foods & Herbs

Alfalfa	Cherries
Anise	Olives
Garlic	Yams
Licorice	Eggplant
Parsley	Tomatoes
Sage	Potatoes
Animal flesh	Pepper
Dairy Food	Cereal grains (except white
Eggs	rice, rye, buckwheat)
Apples	

Although you must vary your diet and eat a wide variety of foods from all of the food groups in order to get as many different nutrients as possible from your food, the following foods should be eaten at intervals rather than daily as many people do. Because of their culture, people tend to eat the kinds of foods they were brought up on. This can be harmful to your well-being during the menopause.

Estrogen Reducing
Foods and Herbs

White rice	Thyme
White flour	Dill
Buckwheat	Onion
Rye	Figs
Tapioca	Pears
Corn	Pineapples
String beans	

Foods that Contribute to
Skin Problems

Shellfish	Iodized salt
Peanut butter	Eggs in large quantities
Organ meats	Steroid fed meat or chicken

Foods that Can Cause
Skin Flushes

Beer, red wine, sherry	Mustard
Spicy foods	Ketchup
Avocados	MSG
Sharp aged cheeses	Processed meats
Caffeinated drinks	Pickled herring
Relish	Nuts

NOTE: It's not that you can't eat any of these foods. However, it's best not to eat them too often. If you notice that any of your symptoms gets worse after eating a particular food, avoid it for a few weeks before adding it back to your menu.

Foods that Tend to Encourage
Water Retention & Bloating

Salt pork	Canned vegetables
Smoked foods	Bacon
Goose	Herring
Bouillon	Soy sauce
Fried foods	Caviar
Duck	Pickles
Gravies	Salted nuts

Foods that Frequently Set off Allergic Reactions

Milk   Tomatoes
Shellfish   Soy
Fish   Pink Peppercorns
Strawberries   Plant foods
Eggs

Foods that Promote Health

Canned salmon   Skim milk
Sardines with bones   Spinach
Yogurt   Kale
Collard greens   Broccoli
Oranges   Almonds
Sesame seeds   Cauliflower

Foods that are Iron-Rich
(However — some are rich in cholesterol)

Pork   Carrots
Lamb   Apricots
Shellfish   Eggs
Spinach   Split peas
Dark meat of the   Chili beans
  turkey and chicken   Lentils
Meat   Squash
Liver   Raisins

If Menopause has Hurt Your Hair and Nails

Salmon	Dried beans
Liver	Nuts
Wheat germ	Fish
Lean beef	Poultry
Yogurt	Eggs
Mushrooms	

Pass the Calcium, Iron, and Zinc

It's hard to be able to judge whether or not you're getting enough of the vital nutrients you need. Supplements are a good form of nutritional insurance. On the following page are some tables which illustrate the mineral content of popular foods. Bear in mind that most of the mineral content *will not* be absorbed.

Zinc Content of Some Foods

Food Item	Serving Size	Mg per serving
Wheat germ	1 tbsp	4.0
Beef, lamb, pork sausages, dark turkey, ham, hamburgers (includes fast foods)	4 oz.	5.0
Liver	2 oz.	3.0
Shellfish, light turkey, dark chicken	3 oz.	2.0
Other fish, light chicken	3 oz.	1.0
Egg	1 egg	0.7
Milk, yogurt, cottage cheese	1 cup	1.2
Cheese	1 oz.	1.0 (1" square)
Legumes	1 cup	0.7
Tofu	1/2 cup	1.0
Nuts, peanuts, peanut butter	1 oz.	0.5
Rice, brown or fortified white	1/2 cup	0.5
Bread, whole wheat, whole grain or fortified cereal**	1 slice	0.5

** The zinc content of cereals varies greatly. Some supply 3 mg per serving. Check the side panel for the amount of zinc per serving supplied by your favorite cereal.

Calcium Content of Some Foods
Source: U.S. Department of Agriculture

Food Item	Serving Size	Mg. per serving
Plain skim and lowfat yogurts	1 cup	350-450
Lowfat flavored and fruited yogurts	1 cup	
Dry nonfat milk	1/4 cup	
Sardines, with bones	3 ounces	
Some fruited yogurts	1 cup	250-350
Skim and lowfat milks	1 cup	
Whole milk, chocolate and buttermilk	1 cup	
Swiss and Gruyere cheeses	1 ounce	
Hard cheeses, Cheddar and Edam	1 ounce	
Processed cheeses	1 ounce	
Cheese spreads	1 ounce	150-250
Salmon, with bones	3 ounces	
Collards	1/2 cup	
Cheese foods	1 ounce	
Soft cheeses, mozzarella, blue, and feta	1 ounce	
Cooked dried beans, navy, pea, and lima	1 cup	
Turnip greens, cale, dandelion greens	1/2 cup	
Ice creams and ice milks	1 ounce	50-150
Evaporated whole milk	1/2 cup	
Cottage cheeses	1/2 cup	
Sherbets	1/2 cup	
Broccoli	1 fresh	
Orange	1/4 cup	
Dates, raisins	1	
Egg	1 slice	
Bread, whole-wheat or white	1/2 cup	
Cabbage	1 ounce	20-50
Cream cheese		

Iron Content of Some Foods

MEAT	Milligrams Per 100 Grams (3.5 oz.)
Beef liver, fried	5.7
Hamburger, cooked, lean	2.7
Lambchop, broiled	1.8
Shrimp	1.8
Chicken breast, roasted	1.04
Perch	0.92
NON-MEAT	
Filberts (hazelnuts)	8.1
Pistachios	6.7
Cashews	6.4
Whole-wheat bread	3.2
Enriched white-bread	3.0
Popcorn (popped with oil)	3.0
White beans (boiled)	3.0
Pinto beans (boiled)	3.0
Chickpeas (boiled)	3.0
Spinach, raw	2.7
Raisins, seeded (Muscat)	2.6
Eggs	2.01
Soybean curd	1.6
Bean sprouts	1.6
Broccoli	1.1
Romaine lettuce	1.1
Avocado	1.0
Iceberg lettuce	0.57
Apple	0.18

Source: U.S. Department of Agriculture

Salads Can Be A Great Help
For The Waistline

Pick the green that helps the most:

Loose leaf lettuces including oat tip and ruby	High in calcium, potassium, vitamin C and vitamin A
Butterhead lettuce	Twice the iron and 3 times as much vitamin C
Spinach	Calcium, potassium, vitamins A and C
Kale	Rich in potassium and calcium, more vitamin A than any other green and 30 times more vitamin C than iceberg lettuce
Turnip and mustard greens	Best for vitamins C and A, best for calcium as well.
Collards	Best for protein and loads of calcium, more vitamin C than iceberg
Beet greens	Twice the iron content of most greens
French sorrel	Great for vitamin A and C, potassium and calcium
Swiss chard	Calcium, vitamin A, iron, potassium

So think twice before you settle for iceberg lettuce and tomato salad. Mix the greens, add some hardboiled eggs, some apple cider vinegar and sunflower or olive oil and pamper yourself while you nourish your nutrient-starved body!

The Exercise Advantage

We've discussed the unwelcome changes menopause brings with it and some of the nutritional efforts that can be made to lesson the impact. Exercise can also curb some of the negative consequences.

Walter M. Borz, II, M.D. and gerontologist, former president of the American Geriatrics Society has stated that many changes commonly attributed to the process of aging are the same changes that accompany physical inactivity.

Therefore, it is possible that some of the discomfort you're feeling may be the result of the "couch potato" state you let yourself fall into. Not all, but let's say 25 percent. So, here's how regular exercise can help you:

* Postmenopausal women become increasing susceptible to coronary artery disease. Exercise helps prevent a decline in high-density-lipoprotein (HDL) and therefore clears cholesterol out of the arteries.

* Exercise also helps the complexion. Older skins tend to dry and lose elasticity. During exercise, the blood flow that carries nutrients and moisture to the facial tissues increases as much as six times over the "couch potato" level.

* Other areas also need the extra moisture. The vaginal area may experience a drying of the mucous membrane. Having regular sex is good exercise. By increasing the blood flow to the vagina, sexual pleasure is maintained.

* Regular exercise leads to better stamina. Lungs, heart and blood vessels will function more effectively.

* As your estrogen level declines so does your ability to metabolize fats. This means more fat is ordinarily put in storage. Regular endurance exercise controls that middle-age spread by helping to burn off fat.

* The thinning and weakening of the bones of the skeletal structure is directly connected to estrogen drop-off. Activity drastically increases the body's ability to utilize calcium. Weight-bearing exercise and stress on the bones helps retard the osteoporotic process by adding bone mass.

* Kegel exercise should be done daily. It is a simple exercise routine in which a woman squeezes and releases the muscles around the vagina and anus 50 to 100 times, three times a day. To find the correct muscles, simply — during urination — stop and start, stop and start. When you can feel which muscles you are using you can practice anywhere. This routine can keep your vaginal area moist and healthy and ward off the incontinence that frequently accompanies aging.

You don't have to go to a gym. Walking, at a reasonable pace, every day is stimulating. Dancing, soft aerobics, even lifting weights is beneficial. Stretching and deep breathing exercises along with a daily walk of a couple of miles is a good beginning.

The Right Vitamins for Women Over 50

About 50 percent of all American women supplement their diet with a multi-vitamin/mineral tablet. That's a good idea because their eating habits and nutrient-depleted food can add up to marginal deficiency. But, are they also taking all that is needed once they hit the menopausal state?

According to a recent study done by the United States Department of Agriculture, Human Nutrition Research Center on Aging, just 26 percent of older women are taking calcium supplements despite the fact that 55 to 75 percent have been shown to be deficient in that key mineral.

Women use vitamin-mineral supplements more than men do, and more older women appreciate their potential to do good for them. While 46 percent of 60 year-olds take supplements, the total rises to 68 percent at age 80.

Despite this widespread use of supplements among older women, good diet has nothing to do with whether or not a person takes them. Frequently, the person with the best diet approach is also the supplement taker. But, after 50, a woman may frequently require different amounts of vitamins and minerals than she did when she was younger. There can be changes in her intestinal tract. For example, as she ages, her ability to absorb calcium decreases. She may need to increase not only the calcium intake but also her intake of vitamin D and vitamin C.

Her ability to taste and appreciate food may decrease due to a problem with zinc. Loneliness can make her limit her meals to tea and toast or anything that she can make easily for herself. Problems with teeth can interfere with efficient digestion and make it more difficult to chew protein-rich foods.

Nutritional surveys indicate that up to two-thirds of women over 50 have vitamin A intakes which are substantially below RDA levels. As the human body ages, both men and women become less able to absorb vitamin B-12 from food. This is especially important for vegetarians because vegetables have no B-12.

Also, as people age they often have a shortage of vitamin C. This may be due to a lack of citrus fruits in the diet which can be corrected. However, since arthritis-like pains are also associated with aging and the use of aspirin for pain depletes the vitamin C content of the body, there may be another good reason to increase the intake of supplemental vitamin C.

Vitamin D may also be on the low level. It can be due to a lack of sunshine because of all the warnings that sunlight can cause skin cancer, cataracts, etc. Sunlight is the causitive agent for the body's production of natural vitamin D. When the sun's rays strike the skin they change cholesterol into another substance that is then made into usable vitamin D. Also, older people tend to drink less milk which is one of the main sources of vitamin D.

Vitamin D and calcium are used together to help treat hot flashes, irritability and depression. Up to 1,500 milligrams of calcium, 400 I.U. of vitamin D and up to 1,000 milligrams of vitamin C daily have been reported as useful in alleviating many of the symptoms.

Even good diets can be low in iron. That fact, coupled with the fact that iron is poorly absorbed from the intestinal tract, makes it easier for women over 50 to suffer from an iron deficiency. Iron supplements plus taking vitamin C along with iron-containing meals and iron supplements can go a long way toward solving the problem.

Zinc is only marginally supplied in the typical American diet. Zinc is tied to hormone levels and a zinc deficiency will influence taste (as said before) as well as the ability to smell succulent aromas of cooking foods. The body prepares itself for digestion long before we sit down to a meal. The lack of the ability to smell and taste food interferes with efficient digestion. Also, because food is tasteless, more salt is used with its bad results on blood pressure. A zinc deficiency can also influence wound healing so that minor wounds take much longer to heal.

Problems at menopause may be more severe because the diet has been deficient in many nutrients for many years prior to its onset. Protein, calcium, magnesium, vitamin D, E, and pantothenic acid, for example. Calcium is less well absorbed and the urinary losses are greater when the output of estrogen decreases. The intake of magnesium should be one-half that of calcium (if you take 1,000 milligrams of calcium then take 500 milligrams of magnesium).

During menopause the need for vitamin E is increased. Hot flashes and night sweats often disappear when 50 to 400 I.U. of vitamin E are taken daily.

Menopausal tension can be eased by taking vitamin A (10,000 to 20,000 I.U. every other day), and the vitamin B-Complex, which helps to normalize blood sugar, destroy excess hormones and soothe nerves. Vitamin E and lecithin help the liver destroy excess hormones and act as natural tranquilizers. Vitamin C helps your body lose water naturally and safely.

It is interesting to note that potassium is an important mineral for proper adrenal function and the adrenals take over when the ovaries shut down. To be completely in balance we should take in twice as much potassium as sodium in our diet. From all of the evidence, our modern diet supplies just the opposite, twice as much sodium as potassium. We may get the correct amount of potassium from food but, if we take in four times as much sodium, it means that the excess sodium forces the body to get rid of the little potassium we take in. Also, diuretics force the excretion of this important mineral. While taking potassium supplements may not be necessary, reducing the sodium intake during menopause is absolutely necessary.

The following table can be a help to figure some of your particular requirements:

<u>Symptom</u>	<u>Vitamins/Daily</u> & <u>Minerals/Daily</u>
Osteoporosis	Vitamins D 400 I.U. Vitamin C 500 mg to 1,000 mg or more. Calcium to 1,500 mg. Magnesium to 750 mg. Boron 3 mg. Manganese 5 mg.
Atherosclerosis	Lecithin 1200 mg/capsule, two with meals. Vitamin E 400 I.U. Vitamin C 1,000 mg. Fish Oil capsules, two with meals.
Irritation and Dryness of Skin and Vaginal Area	Vitamin A 10,1000 I.U.
Hot Flashes	Vitamin E 400 I.U.
Emotional Problems	Vitamin B-Complex 50 mg L-tryptophan 500 mg.
Psychological Problems	L-Phenylalanine or L-Tyrosine 500 mg

Along with this, you have to change your diet and lifestyle.

Do regular exercises daily and try to get ten minutes of sunlight a day. Eat canned sardines, milk and milk products, salmon, green vegetables, sesame seeds, fish, garlic, sunflower seeds, liver, eggs, carrot juice and use cold-pressed vegetable oils.

Avoid smoking, alcohol, caffeine, excess meats, aluminum-containing antacids.

Dr. Stuart M. Berger, M.D., in his book, *How To Be Your Own Nutritionist*, Avon Books, N.Y., considers the following to be necessary:

Vitamin B-Complex	1 tablet daily
Vitamin D	400 I.U.
Vitamin E	600 I.U.
Selenium	150 micrograms
Calcium	1,500 mg
Magnesium	1,000 mg

Paavo Airola, Ph.D., in his book, *How To Get Well*, recommends:

Vitamin E	up to 1,200 I.U.
Vitamin B-6	up to 100 mg
Brewer's yeast	3 to 4 tbsp.
Vitamin A	50,000 I.U.
Vitamin B-1	50 mg
Calcium lactate	3 tablets
PABA	up to 100 mg
B-Complex	1 tablet
Pantothenic acid	up to 100 mg
Kelp	up to 3 tablets daily
Whey powder	2 tsp.
Vitamin C	up to 3,000 mg
Cod Liver Oil	2 tsp. or 4 capsules

Cold-pressed oil such as sesame or olive oil.

Juices freshly made of fruits and vegetables in season.

Herbs, sarsaparilla, licorice, unicorn root, because they contain natural estrogen to help compensate for the diminished supply in the body.

Homeopathy: A Likely, Natural Alternative

Homeopathy is a branch of medicine which views the menopause in a fundamentally different way from the currently popular and conventional allopathic approach. Homeopathic treatment itself is different. Very small doses of natural drugs, which are completely safe, are prescribed.

Basically, the philosophy is that like treats like. In other words, the menopause is treated with a remedy that has the ability to produce in a healthy person symptoms that are similar to those observed now in the patient.

Homeopathy has been part of medical practice for centuries. It was known to the ancient Greeks. Hippocrates wrote of symptoms as the expression of nature's healing powers. The founder of modern homeopathy is generally acknowledged to be Samuel Hahnemann.

The theory behind homeopathy is similar to the principle of vaccines. Vaccines operate on the logic that "like prevents like," and are actually small doses of the very disease they are trying to prevent. The disease is introduced into the body so that the immune system may build up a tolerance and combat it if the toxin intrudes on a large scale. That idea, in homeopathy, is simply extended to "like cures like."

If there is any rule to be followed, it is not to use any stimulating or aromatic substances including garlic, mint, camphor, caffeine, tobacco, or even spicy foods immediately before or after taking a remedy. They can interfere with any beneficial effects.

Although there have not been any double-blind research studies confirming the value of homeopathy in treating the symptoms of menopause, there is pragmatic clinical experience which shows relief of syptoms when the remedies are utilized. Also, they cannot hurt.

Some of the common remedies are Sepia and Natrummur. The other commonly used remedy is called Lachesis. Other common medicines for the menopausal symptoms are Calcarea carbonica, sulphur, and less frequently, Apis, Graphites, Phosphorus, and Psorinum.

Hemopathic physicians are usually to be found in all of the states. Use of the remedies plus diet and exercise can answer all of your problems. However, it's not necessary to go to a physician to try these remedies. Drug stores and health food stores have specific remedies that you can buy over the counter.

A Menopause Diet

A good diet high in low-stress foods can help you get through the worst of it.

The 25 best low-stress foods are:

Sprouts, whole grain cereals and breads, fish, beans, lowfat milk, lean poultry, raw seeds and nuts, tropical fruits, yogurt, citrus fruits, bran and wheat germ, garlic, oats, brown rice, sea vegetables and dark green leafy vegetables, root vegetables, tofu, herb tea and the use of cold-pressed vegetable oil.

If you know what's best for you, you should also be aware of the worst:

Salt, bacon, french fries, soft drinks, regular tea, fatty beef, pork sausages, coffee, pie, cake, salted pickles, chocolate, salted snacks, soup mixes, canned food of all kinds, non-dairy creamers, white sugar, white flour, animal shortenings, margarine, deep-fried anything, full fat cheese, excess meat, fast foods.

Here are some general diet concepts which will serve your body well during the trying times and also will keep you on your toes from then on:

Breakfast:
Try to have one fresh fruit and one dried fruit. Prunes with a fruit juice daily will help to keep you regular.

Herbal tea.

Oatmeal, cornmeal, Muesli, millet. Try to have a variety of cereals during the week.

Eggs should be hardboiled.

Lunch:
Salads every day.
Make dressings of avocado, cheese and yogurt, nut butter, olive oil and apple cider vinegar.
Vegetables. Try to use one above-ground vegetable and one root vegetable.
Brown rice, baked potato, lima beans, yams.

Dinner:
Meat no more than three times a week, lean, no fat, no pork.
Use chicken, turkey, beef, meatloaf, fish.
Two cooked vegetables and a salad.
Twice a week have a vegetarian meal.

Natural Alternatives

Beet Juice
A combination of beet juice and carrot juice (using roots and tops) made by using from 3 to 8 ounces of beet juice to a pint of the combination, has been very helpful in alleviating some of the menopausal symptoms.

Taken alone, beet juice, in greater quantities than a wineglass at a time, may cause a cleansing reaction which can make a person a little dizzy or nauseated. Therefore, the combination with carrot juice is recommended.

Dong Quai
This Chinese herb is helpful in correcting hot flashes and spasms of the vagina. It has also been reported to be amazingly effective in cases of menopausal rheumatism.

Capsules containing Dong Quai in powdered form are available in health food stores. The capsules may be swallowed with a glass of warm water or broken open and the contents added to hot soups or broths. Chinese herbalists advise that fruit should not be eaten for at least three hours before or after taking this herb. Vegetables can and should be eaten along with Dong Quai.

(From, *Secrets of the Chinese Herbalists*, Richard Lucas, Reward Books, Parker Pub. Co., West Nyack, N.Y.)

Lecithin

Lecithin affects the transmission of nerve messages having to do with sexuality and the endocrine glands. All systems need lecithin to function but during menopause, the sexual system is in the greatest need. Get lecithin capsules, 1200 milligrams each or Phos-Cal capsules (more concentrated but also more expensive). Your health food store will have them in stock. Take two capsules with meals.

Garlic

Garlic has been used since earliest times. It is a natural antiseptic, a tonic to the lymphatic system, and it offers soothing relief to the bladder. It helps to balance the endocrine glands and helps to restore the body's balance during menopause.

Herbal Teas

Herbal preparations are milder, safer and, because they are like foods, may take longer to have an observable effect. But, they also have fewer side effects than prescription medicines. You can use a capsule to make tea or, if you prefer, make tea from the roots, leaves or bark. If you're using roots, leaves, bark, etc., take a tablespoon of the mixture and add it to one cup of water in a stainless steel saucepan. Bring to a boil for 15 minutes. Let it cool for five minutes. Strain and sip. You can add honey as a sweetener if you desire.

Black Cohosh

Contains a natural estrogen. Helps to relieve cramps.

Black Hawthorne

Eases cramps and uterine congestion.

Blessed Thistle

Can be used for same symptoms.

Echinacea
Tonic to the reproductive system.

False Unicorn
Tones uterus.

Fo-ti-Tien
Endocrine gland rejuvenation.

Ginseng
Stimulates hormone production.

Gotu Kola
Similar properties to ginseng.

Licorice
Do not use if you have high blood pressure. Stimulates female glands, stimulates the adrenal cortex. Can be used with ginseng and sarsaparilla.

Oat Straw
Aids in uterine and ovarian disorders.

Red Raspberry
Strengthens female reproductive system.

Sarsaparilla
Contains hormone-like compounds beneficial to the sexual system.

Saw Palmetto
Helps balance hormone levels.

Squaw Vine
Can work marvels for cramps — especially menstrual and menopausal cramps.

This is a sampling of herbs. Your health food store will have individual herbs or herbal combinations combined for your use by manufacturers. Most stores have books or pamphlets to help you choose the herb best suited to your symptoms.

Passiflora, Viburnum opulus and cimicifuga appear in many herbal formulas, although not listed here. That is because herbal remedies follow different traditions. Some formulas are from Chinese sources, some from Indian sources and some from Tibetan sources. Our Native Americans used these herbs. Most formulas have a long tradition of satisfaction behind them but you will have to try several to find the formulas that suit you the best.

Dong Quai (Tang kwai) is often taken in combination with other herbs such as peony, rehmannia and licorice. Since you cannot easily find the raw materials, it is better to rely on the prepared combination in capsule form which can be made into a tea.

Suma

Suma is a South American herb used as a strengthening tonic for women and as an adaptogenic herb by herbalists. An adaptogenic is a substance that does not harm the body but, by working through the hormones, helps the body adapt to stress. The active ingredients in Suma are called saponins; specifically, pfaffosides, which are water soluble and make a beneficial, strengthening and regulating tea.

Vitex (Vitex agnus-castus)

These are berries of a small shrub from Europe. They appear to work with the glands in helping conditions called fibroid cysts and menopausal symptoms. Your store may have capsules of Vitex under the name of Chaste Tree.

Ginger

Hot ginger tea can work marvels for cramps. It's usually found in combination with other herbs in your health food store but you can make your own by adding a small amount of fresh ginger to a cup of boiling water and letting it simmer for ten minutes. Let cool, strain and add some honey to taste.

L-Phenylalanine & L-Tryosine
These amino acids (found especially in meat and cheese) are precursors of (chemically converted to) norepinephrine, the brain's version of adrenalin, and also dopamine. The depression associated with menopause may respond to the use of either amino acid. They come in 500 milligram tablets or capsules and one capsule can be of great help. If you suffer from any form of high blood pressure try L-Tyrosine instead of L-Phenylalanine. In any event, check with your doctor first, especially if you are on any type of medication.

L-Tryptophan
An amino acid which has been very useful in helping to restore normal sleep patterns when taken at night and alleviating anxiety when taken during the day. It can be found in health food stores in tablet or capsule form, usually in a 500 milligram dose. You can take one or two at night with a glass of milk or a cookie to help you sleep. If you find that you are anxious during the day you may want to take one tablet or capsule. However, since it may make you drowsy, don't drive, operate or be around heavy machinery. In any event, check first with your doctor, especially if you are taking any medication.

Clinical Studies

There have been very few clinical studies done on menopausal symptoms. Here are some of the most relevant:

Chicago Med., March 7, 1964
Bioflavonoids (citrus derived) were much more effective than sub-therapeutic doses of estrogens and 2 other treatments which have been suggested in non-hormonal control of vaso-motor flushing in menopausal patients.

New York State Medical Journal, May 15, 1952, 00. 1289-91
Vitamin E 100 mg. 3 times daily cured menopausal symptoms within three months.

Ann. West. Med. & Surg., 4 (1):27-32, 1950

In a preliminary study, 37 out of 59 patients with hot flashes and sweats, 16 out of 28 with backaches and muscle pains, and 16 out of 34 with menorrhagia improved on 10 to 25 mg. of vitamin E daily. Seventy-nine additional patients received either 50 or 100 mg vitamin E daily. At least 75 percent of patients with hot flashes and sweats improved and up to 86 percent were relieved of backaches, joint pains and headaches within 4 weeks.

11 out of 12 patients with dizziness, 9 out of 11 with palpitations, and 3 out of 4 with dyspnea were relieved within 2 weeks. Up to 70 percent of patients with fatigue and 67 percent of patients with nervousness were relieved within 8 weeks.

J. Clin. Endocrin. Metabol., 9:89-94, 1949

66 patients with vasomotor symptoms were given vitamin E for 10 days to 7 months (ave. 31 days). 31 had good to excellent results and 16 had fair results with prompt recurrence of symptoms after discontinuation of the vitamin.

American Journal Obstet. & Gyn., 50:84, 1945

25 women with intractable hot flashes and a history of cancer which made estrogen supplementation inappropriate received 10 to 30 mg of vitamin E daily for 1 to 6 weeks. All responded with either complete relief or marked improvement of hot flashes and they reported positive mood changes. There were no untoward side effects.

British Medical Journal, 1:242-3, 1976

A positive correlation was found between low blood levels of tryptophan and estrogen in depressed women who had gone through menopause. Deficiency may be associated with menopausal depression.

NUTRITIONAL ENGINEERING

How To Keep Your Bad Habits

... And Still Avoid Flame-out

by David A. Keiper

Bad Habits

Have you ever wondered how some people seem to get away with all kinds of bad habits? Are they really getting away with high living, or will there be a later reckoning? A few may get off scot-free — those who have inherited an iron constitution. But for us ordinary mortals, is there a way that we can extend our usual limits? There certainly is. We can achieve optimum health — a state in which our body is best able to withstand all the insults thrown at it, whether they come from bad habits, stress, or exposure to environmental pollutants.

In the case of men, modern medicine has failed them. American men now die more than seven years younger than women, on average, and male "bad habits" are blamed for much of the sizable difference in life expectancy. Some habits widely believed to be "bad" are relatively benign and you can do some nutritional engineering to protect yourself.

The one habit you can't get away with is the modern civilized diet. It is much worse than the worst of the usual "bad habits", but most likely, you'll be pleasantly surprised with the modest dietary changes you need. Many nutritionists mistakenly lay a bum rap on foods containing fat and cholesterol and that allows some worse culprits to go unchecked. Also, men have somewhat different nutritional needs than women, but few nutritionists seem to appreciate the full extent of the differences.

Complicating the story are vast genetic differences between individuals. This is especially true of our nutritional needs. Thus you must ultimately become the expert on your own body and its needs.

On all sides, people have been telling you that you have to give up smoking, drinking, type "A" behavior, trim your weight down, get more exercise, or quit eating certain foods that have fat, cholesterol, salt, or sugar in them. Others tell you to watch out for the additives, preservatives, or pesticides in your food. Still other experts warn you about the air you breathe and the water you drink. At any time now you expect some expert to come out with: "Warning! Living may be hazardous to your health."

The implied threat, if you ignore their warnings, is that you may suffer *flame-out*. A flame-out is always much more serious, dramatic and sudden than a "burn-out", and can involve a loss of life, loss of control over life, or just a serious loss of self-esteem. Men are far more likely to flame-out than women.

A common way to flame-out is by a heart attack. Or another type of flame-out (reserved for men) is sexual impotence — a depressing experience, but not fatal.

With so many of our habits alleged to be bad by a variety of experts, how are we going to sort out which expert to listen to?

Sometimes the experts contradict one another, and sometimes the facts contradict the experts.

1. Smoking is considered an important risk factor in male heart disease. Yet in Greece, where there is a low rate of coronary heart disease, and where the 45-year old male has a higher life expectancy than in any other country, men smoke the most cigarettes.

2. Exercise has been touted as a protection against heart disease. However, we hear of experienced marathoners dropping dead of a heart attack.

3. Cholesterol has become the equivalent of the "bogeyman" in some circles. In ignorant fear, many fail to make the distinction between *dietary* cholesterol (found in some of our most nutritious foods) and *blood* cholesterol level. When the blood serum level of cholesterol is elevated above normal for a period of many years, there is an increased risk of coronary heart disease. Most of the cholesterol in your bloodstream is manufactured by your own body, so the problem of an elevated blood cholesterol level is primarily a problem of the body's regulation of it rather than one of dietary intake.

4. Food fat is considered a major contributor to heart disease when consumed in excess. However, the Masai tribesmen of East Africa, for example, take in a whopping 65 percent of their calories in food fat, mostly saturated, but have almost no heart disease at any age.

5. The idea of stress (type "A" behavior) as a cause of heart disease is continuing to grow in popularity. Stress is undoubtedly an important contributing factor in many cases, but can't be the whole story, since unstressed (type "B") individuals get heart attacks, too.

The key to understanding it all depends upon appreciating the many *interactions* that occur between the "bad habit" factors and certain nutritional factors. The field of nutritional biochemistry is a vast and rapidly growing body of knowledge published in reputable biological-medical journals. While conventional thinking can never hope to make good progress against coronary heart disease, nutritional biochemical approaches may get close to eradicating it because there is good evidence that the modern civilized diet is a major cause — although a delayed cause — of heart attacks.

You need to switch from fluid milk to yogurt and cheese, and from refined grains and sugars to whole grains and starches. You also need more sources of omega-3 oil — often called "EPA" or "fish oil," but which is also available from certain vegetable sources. As additional protection, you may need more vegetables and salads, and to ease off a bit on salt and fat — advisable especially for those who have a family history of heart disease. Following this advice, I estimate you can reduce your chances of a heart attack by 90 percent. If you add on vitamin and mineral supplementation tailored to individual needs, the chances would be reduced by 99 percent.

It appears that we have been brainwashed to believe in the importance of the conventional risk factors like eggs, red meat, smoking, and drinking, when actually the main heart risks are in certain aspects of the modern civilized diet that were not fully appreciated.

Helping Men Live Longer

It's the quality of life that most concerns us, not the years lived. Yet what popular type of drug is used to lower high blood pressure or prevent a second heart attack? It's called a "beta-blocker" and it subdues your reaction to outside stimuli. As a side effect, some men will lose interest in sex or be unable to get an erection. What man wants this sort of drug approach for extending his life? Certainly, life would seem longer.

One key to increasing male life expectancy, and improving the quality of life in the later years, lies in raising male consciousness of the importance of certain nutritional factors. (Wives/mates can help here.)

Nutritional therapy — improving/modifying the diet and using vitamin and mineral supplements — can help far more than drugs. Nutritional therapy has few adverse side effects. In fact, it frequently has beneficial side effects, like curing more health problems than the therapist set out to cure.

As an example of how nutritional therapy can save lives, consider some research work of James P. Isaacs, M.D. He had available 25 people who had one or more heart attacks and who were failing under the conventional cardiology treatment of the 1960's. He gave them balanced nutritional supplements which included both vitamins and minerals. (Also included was a modest dose of thyroid hormone.)

Of the 21 men in the program, 19 were alive and well 10 years later and had no further heart attacks. Of the two men lost, one died soon after the program began, when he returned too quickly to a job that required physical exertion. The other quit the supplements after six years, developed angina, and then died of a heart attack while doctors were using invasive procedures to examine his arteries. Perhaps both deaths were unnecessary, and would not happen today with the latest knowledge of both nutritional therapy and conventional cardiology treatment. It indicates how much the coronary patient's life can hang in the balance and be tipped over by small events.

The 90% survival rate for the men in Isaac's study was remarkable, especially considering the fact that the patients were chosen because they were failing after their heart attacks. During the nutritional therapy, the men had other health improvements, such as greater exercise tolerance, better skin texture and appearance, reduced problems with teeth and gums, etc. All symptoms of heart disease disappeared. If nutritional therapy had not been used, probably less than half the men would have survived, and the survivors might have led a rather limited life.

For comparison, let us look at the results of various drug trials in some rather expensive research projects. Results in 1981 showed that beta-blocking drugs can reduce the incidence of second heart attacks by 30%. In 1984, it was shown that a drug that lowers blood cholesterol could reduce heart attacks 20% in *high risk* males. I emphasize "high risk" because it won't necessarily do anything for the average male. Besides, among the men getting the drug, there was an alarming number of men dying in accidents or suicide, or developing cancer.

In late 1987, the drug gemfibrozil was shown to reduce heart disease rates by one-third in high risk males. In early 1988, results were released showing that one aspirin tablet every other day reduces the heart attack rate by 47% in middle-aged male physicians, apparently by reducing blood-platelet aggregation and thus the tendency for blood clots to form in the coronary arteries.

However, not widely addressed are aspirin's many side effects, including an increased risk of bleeding into the brain, leading to a stroke. There are instead certain nutritional factors that contribute to normalizing excessive blood-platelet aggregation. Because of risks of serious side effects, it doesn't seem to make much sense to take aspirin or the other drugs.

The comparable figure on the reduction of second heart attacks through nutritional therapy, based upon Dr. Isaacs work, would be 80% (or higher, depending upon how the data is handled). On top of that, nutritional therapy had beneficial side effects, whereas the drug therapies had annoying side effects and the latest nutritional therapy, individualized for the patient and carried out by an M.D. of the nutritional specialty, could virtually eliminate second heart attacks.

If nutritional therapy can cure heart trouble in those who have already had a heart attack, it should certainly be able to prevent heart attacks in those who have never had one. The vitamin and mineral lackings most often implicated in Western Coronary Heart Diseases are: vitamin C, vitamin E, vitamin B-6, omega-3 oil, magnesium, potassium, selenium, chromium, copper, and zinc, so prevention is certainly the best strategy. It only requires modest changes in diet, plus the use of vitamin and mineral supplements: vitamin C, vitamin E, vitamin B-6, magnesium, omega-3 oil, and substances in pineapple (bromelin), garlic and onions.

Staying Out Of Trouble

Of course, everyone extols prevention. But we don't practice it often. One of the major reasons may be that we have difficulty perceiving a cause-effect relationship when the effect lags the cause by time periods greater than a few days.

Another hindrance to the practice of prevention is the illusion of invincibility, probably more a problem with men than women. I am no better than the rest of you. At one time, I had a dozen different annoying health complaints, and blindly missed seeing the connections between biochemistry and the food going into my mouth.

A friend happened to toss a nutrition book at me and, over a period of many years of study, I managed to eliminate most of my health problems through improved diet.

Over the same span of time, the field of nutritional therapy has also been developing. Along the way, I met many other people who had been let down by conventional medical practice, and found that many of them could also be helped by nutritional therapy. It is unfortunate that doctors get very little training in nutrition in medical school. Thus they miss out on some of the better ways of helping many of their patients.

Also working against the practice of prevention are the addictions that we acquire to the many readily available taste-tempting treats and seductive sweets. Surprisingly, some of the foods to which we get addicted are ones that we are allergic to.

Another hindrance to prevention is a fatalistic argument that we sometimes hear. Let's say that your father and your grandfather died young of heart disease. Thus you fully expect to do the same, and think that there is nothing you can do about it. Totally wrong! There are probably a number of different genetic factors that raise susceptibility to coronary heart disease, but all should be treatable by specific nutritional therapies. If you are at risk, it is all the more reason to be nutritionally cautious. Superior nutrition and the right vitamin and mineral supplements will help protect you from disability or an early grave.

A further important hindrance to the practice of prevention is that a heart attack can seem to strike with no warning at all. Don't forget that only about sixty percent of those who have a heart attack get a chance to correct their nutrition. The other forty percent end up on a slab at the coroner's.

The message is: You can keep your own heart in good repair by providing it with all the nutritional factors it needs. Then you'll probably never need medical heroics like coronary bypass, balloon angioplasty, clot-dissolving drugs, etc., practiced on you.

Dietary Drift

Let us look at the drastic changes that have occurred in the American diet since 1860. In 1860, the average American diet, based upon percent of calories, was 12% protein, 25% fat, 53% complex carbohydrates (starches), and 10% simple carbohydrates (sugars). Now the diet is 12-15% protein, 40-45% fat, 22% complex carbohydrates, and 24% simple carbohydrates. There have been drastic increases in fats and sugars, both of which are nutrient-poor fragments of food, and drastic decreases in consumption of nutrient rich starches, such as potatoes and grains.

Furthermore, most of the grains these days have had their germ and bran (fiber) removed. In effect, many of the most heart-protective nutrients have been stripped from the food supply. These include macro-nutrients like vitamin E, omega-3 oil, magnesium and potassium. Only a fraction of the trace elements found in primitive diets survived. Lost were much of the six trace elements that appear protective of the heart and circulatory system: chromium, selenium, zinc, copper, manganese, and silicon.

Around 1920, when the rate of coronary heart disease was rising fast and first becoming significant, magnesium, vitamin B-6, vitamin E, and trace element intakes were in a steady downward trend. Increasing steadily at that time were the intakes of fat and milk. Milk became more popular perhaps because pasteurization made milk much safer from bacterial contamination. Milk is a major source of calcium. Vitamin D was discovered and later became popular in the form of cod liver oil. No doubt, the trend toward calcium and vitamin D helped decrease strokes. But all of the trends were adverse to heart health.

After World War II, we experienced sharp increases in coronary heart disease. At that time, there were sharply increasing intakes of sodium, calcium, and vitamin D. Total fat consumption was rising steadily. All of these trends worked against heart health.

Coronary heart disease peaked in the 1960's. It is rather curious that the two nutrient ratios of calcium to magnesium, and of sodium to potassium also peaked about that time.

Interestingly, total fat consumption has continued its inexorable rise after coronary heart disease peaked, a fact that helps let total fat off the hook as far as being a direct cause. Saturated animal fat consumption did not increase during this century, so it can not be a major cause.

In the 1960's and 1970's some Americans began taking vitamin pills in earnest. Curiously, the decrease in coronary heart disease since the 1960's matches well to the consumption of vitamin C and the idea of a connection is really not so far-fetched, for even mild scurvy tends to promote sudden cardiac death. The movement toward whole foods and taking vitamins caught on first in California, and that is where heart deaths first started decreasing. However, because heart disease rates were decreasing in several other Western countries that didn't experience the vitamin pill-popping fad, it is likely that dietary changes were more important than vitamin pills in the earlier phase of the decreases in coronary heart disease.

There is a wide diversity in the diets of the more developed countries, and a wide diversity in the rates of coronary heart disease. Some years ago, several separate groups of researchers noticed that the rate of coronary heart disease went up with the dietary ratio of calcium to magnesium. An exception were the Masai of East Africa, who also have the highest intake of cholesterol and saturated animal fat in the world, yet have virtually no coronary heart disease and only a minimum of atherosclerotic plaque in old age. There are two protective dietary factors here. They do not use sodium chloride at all, so their dietary sodium-to-potassium ratio is extremely low and they are also the world's greatest partakers of yogurt.

The Masai type of diet is not unique. The Tibetan nomads live on a high plateau (altitude 15,000 to 18,000 feet) about 300 miles North of Lhasa and most of their diet comes from their yak herds.

They eat yak meat, drink yak milk, and eat yak yogurt and butter. Although they consume a small amount of grains, they have no fruits or vegetables. They drink tea with yak butter and salt in it. In spite of this high fat and cholesterol diet, there is no evidence of high blood pressure or heart disease among them. There appears to be a "threshold" level of fermented milk consumption, a level above which there is a significantly lower rate of coronary heart disease. That level would be about 9 to 10 g/day milk protein, or about one cup of yogurt or 1.5 oz. of cheese.

Two countries, Japan and Portugal, happen to have the world's highest rate of stroke deaths in middle-aged males. Both countries also have extremely high dietary ratios of sodium to potassium, no doubt from their consumption of salted fish. In contrast, the Masai have the lowest ratio, and all the other Western countries have sodium-to-potassium ratios in between. Therefore, we can conclude that the sodium-to-potassium ratio is likely to be important in coronary heart disease, as well as in strokes.

Fat consumption does not appear so important, since the countries with the highest fat consumption only have slightly more coronary heart disease than expected from the calcium-to-magnesium ratio. Because high fat diets are generally low nutrient-density diets in Western countries, the lack of nutrients could be the more important contributor to heart disease. A low nutrient-density diet could make one's body unable to handle fat properly.

The key factors appear to be high dietary ratios of calcium to magnesium, and sodium to potassium. An important protective factor would be the consumption of fermented milk products — cheese and yogurt. A minor adverse factor would be total fat consumption. If we had the data from all the world's countries, we would likely find that *all* countries fit into this scheme. Calcium consumption in Western countries is very much a function of the intake of milk and its products; whereas magnesium consumption is very much a function of dietary whole-complex-carbohydrates (whole grains and vegetables). Thus the dietary ratio of calcium to magnesium will go up most in a diet featuring milk and refined foods (refined grains and sugar). Milk by itself has ten times as much calcium as magnesium. The presence of other foods in the diet will bring the ratio down to the usual range of one to four. The ratio also depends somewhat on the sources of animal protein in the diet; thus the consumption of red meats raises the ratio slightly, fish lowers it a bit, and fowl has a neutral effect.

Obviously, the all-American he-man diet is the worst, containing the least magnesium. But magnesium is not the only protective nutrient found in whole foods. Some others are vitamin E, omega-3 oil, vitamin B-6, trace elements and fiber — mostly lost through refinement. Both fiber and yogurt are apt to be protective by improving intestinal functioning.

From what I've said so far about electrolyte mineral ratios, it would appear that both calcium and sodium are bad actors in the matter of heart attacks. But it turns out that calcium shows a highly protective effect as to high blood pressure and strokes. Thus, the Western countries with the lowest stroke rates take in over 1000 milligrams per day of calcium, and countries with the highest stroke rates take in only about 500 mg/day. Are we then forced to make a choice between having a stroke and having a heart attack? I think not.

To see this, we have to consider that in the least developed countries, the calcium intake is certainly no more than 500 mg/day, and that neither high blood pressure nor strokes tend to occur. In these countries, the people do not use salt — in fact, there is no word for salt in the Masai language. From their whole foods, people of the Third World take in generous amounts of potassium (and magnesium, trace elements, omega-3 oil, etc.).

There is recent strong evidence that excess salt, or a high sodium-to-potassium ratio, causes a loss of calcium through the urine, and hence an increase in the calcium requirements. When those high calcium requirements are met by use of milk, Western peoples are put at risk of heart attacks. However, there appears to be a way out of the apparent dilemma. If you consume whole grains and vegetables, your ratios of sodium-to-potassium and calcium-to-magnesium will both be low, and you should not be at risk of either stroke or heart attack. Those people who are genetically salt-sensitive will probably need to hold down their sodium intake as well.

The optimum ratio of calcium to magnesium in the diet for individuals may be somewhere in the range of 1.5 to 1.8. Curiously, the World Health Organization (W. H. O.) suggests a calcium-to-magnesium ratio of about 1.0, whereas the U.S. Recommended Dietary Allowance (RDA) recommends a ratio of 2.3 (calcium 800 and magnesium 350 mg. per day). The W. H. O. figure appears too low, and the U.S. RDA appears too high. Thus it seems that the U.S. RDA has built into it a substantial rate of male heart deaths. But again, it depends upon the intakes of salt and cheese or yogurt.

Research does not have the final answers as yet. Even if a full explanation is not possible at this time, it is clear what dietary changes we have to make. Of importance to commercial interests is the fact that the needed changes don't affect our basic food supply, but only require changes in food processing; that is, milk must be processed more and grains less, and less salt must be added during food processing.

The rate of coronary heart disease in women is much lower than that for men, and there is a greater chance for other factors to be important. Smoking may be the #1 risk factor in women, but in men the dietary drift during the past century is apt to be #1. In males, the hormone testosterone no doubt contributes to the higher rates of coronary heart disease, acting in synergy with dietary drift. Of course, women have testosterone too, but the levels in women are a good bit lower.

More About Minerals

The body can tolerate a certain amount of imbalance in the diet without adverse effects, by regulating absorption from the gut, by kidney retention, by fecal excretion, or even by perspiration. Blood serum levels of the electrolyte minerals are fairly carefully regulated, but magnesium appears to be the least well regulated. The body's normal reaction to stress knocks magnesium out of action. Magnesium is lost through the kidneys by either alcohol or sugar consumption. Body stores of magnesium can easily get depleted, especially in consumers of the all-American low-magnesium diet.

In the human diet, whole grains and vegetables are a main source of magnesium, but these have many more protective factors in them than just magnesium. Vitamin E could be an important one, but omega-3 oil, trace elements, fiber, and vitamin B-6 could be others.

Thus I do not suggest taking just magnesium supplements, for it would be far safer to get magnesium plus all the other protective factors in whole grains and vegetables. When hard water contains significant magnesium, there is a higher concentration of magnesium in people's heart muscles, and lower death rates from coronary heart disease, with fewer of the deaths being sudden.

Water that is hard with magnesium is able to significantly lower the overall dietary calcium-to-magnesium ratio in localities where the people tend to have a low intake of food magnesium.

Inside the body, magnesium deficiency has numerous adverse effects. It promotes atherosclerosis, spasms of the coronary arteries, blood clots (thrombosis), and loss of magnesium by the heart muscle cells. Coronary artery spasms often lead to angina pectoris (chest pains). There is a tendency for heart muscle cells to get selectively depleted of magnesium, while other of the body's muscle cells manage to hang on to their magnesium. The higher rate of metabolism in heart muscle cells probably contributes to this effect.

Magnesium is really a key electrolyte because it helps to regulate the other electrolyte minerals — calcium, sodium, and potassium. Magnesium helps keep the "ion pump" in cell membranes working properly, i.e., pumping sodium ions out of the cells, which helps to hold potassium ions in the cells.

The production of energy within the heart muscle cells is dependent upon adequate magnesium. This energy is ultimately transformed into mechanical work through heart muscle cell contraction and the resultant pumping of blood.

Magnesium also helps maintain normal electrical potentials on the surface of heart muscle cells. This is all important for transmission of the electrical impulses that trigger heart muscle cell contraction. An irregular heart beat (called arrhythmia) is a frequent result of magnesium depletion.

A magnesium lack relates to a far more deadly form of irregular heart beat — ventricular fibrillation, which is a rapid and chaotic contraction of heart muscle cells. Unless interrupted by an electric shock to the chest, or possibly by beating on the chest, death occurs in minutes. Ventricular fibrillation is most likely to happen when there is a sudden change in oxygen supply to the heart, whether up or down.

The gradual development of atherosclerosis produces a slow decrease in oxygen supply to the heart. This more steady oxygen shortage causes the heart muscle cells to lose magnesium, thus interfering with both the ion pump and energy production. As the situation continues to deteriorate, the heart muscle loses potassium and gains sodium and calcium.

At the same time, the normal heart muscle fuel (fatty acids) can't be utilized efficiently, causing further waste of oxygen that is already in short supply. At this point, normal everyday stresses could cause damage to the heart muscle cells, and even mild exercise could do it. Because stress itself can cause further magnesium loss, a vicious circle can be set into motion. The result can be self-destruction of part of the heart muscle. This is euphemistically called a coronary event.

In heart muscle cells, the loss of magnesium and potassium, and the gain of sodium and calcium, is a general disorder that occurs in various forms of heart disease, including coronary atherosclerosis, heart enlargement, congestive heart failure, heart attack, and sudden cardiac death.

As a research experiment, I obtained from the local coroner samples of hair from middle-aged men who had died of sudden cardiac death. An assay of the hair minerals revealed a unique pattern of levels among the minerals calcium, sodium and potassium. The pattern suggested electrolyte derangement in three out of eight men. Two other men showed toxic levels of lead in the hair, which is often evidence of too low a dietary intake of calcium, magnesium and trace minerals. Thus 62% showed evidence of mineral imbalances being behind sudden cardiac death.

Considering all the various data, it is apparent that electrolyte derangement has to be recognized as a major factor in coronary heart disease. I have no doubt that it results directly from dietary mineral imbalances, most likely from a low magnesium intake, with possible contributions from other nutrient deficiencies or excesses, from pollutants, or even from bad habits.

The Sacred Cow

In recent years, there has been a large milk surplus. We can expect the advertising campaigns from the milk industry to continue, but the dairy industry should advertise yogurt and cheese more, and lay off pushing milk because of the many health problems it creates. In fairness, I have to add that the hazards of milk tend to become manifest when there are appreciable refined carbohydrates in the diet.

Of all foods, milk produces the most problems — lactose intolerance, allergies and hypersensitivities. Lactose intolerance is a genetic trait in which an enzyme that digests milk sugar is missing from the gut. Milk then brings on diarrhea or other GI complaints. Usually the individuals affected can tolerate small amounts of milk. Lactose intolerance is experienced by 95% of Orientals; 70% of Blacks; 67% of peoples of Jewish heritage or of Eastern or Central Europe or Mediterranean origins; and 18% of whites in the U. S. A.

Milk allergy can lead to a variety of different symptoms, ranging from subtle to cataclysmic, which usually occur about a half-hour after ingestion. If your pulse rate climbs above 85 (normal being about 70) a half-hour after consuming milk, it is a good clue that you have a milk allergy.

Hypersensitivities to milk can be varied and subtle, and appear hours or days after ingestion. One of the most common symptoms is stuffy sinuses. Even small quantities can get a big reaction. In some men, it appears connected to aggressiveness or violence. [McGee '79]

As to milk's connection to coronary disease, there is some intriguing evidence:

People who have lactose intolerance tend to stay away from milk, and thus have much less coronary heart disease.

Men on a milk diet for ulcers have more than twice as many heart attacks on average as ulcer patients on an ordinary diet.

In Japan, milk consumption went up by a factor of ten over the past 30 years, which is a far greater change than for any other food. Over the same period, the rate of coronary heart disease went up, and that of strokes went down. Older men seemed to be most affected.

In Switzerland, a 22% decrease in male coronary heart disease occurred over a 25 year period during which milk consumption decreased 46%.

In the U. S. A., since the 1960's, there has been a strong movement away from milk, and toward cheese and yogurt. During this period the death rate from coronary heart disease has decreased about 30%.

In all statistical correlations, milk is the food most associated with coronary heart disease. The damaging effect is strongest for unfermented milk, with a protective effect seen in fermented milk — cheese or yogurt. Since fermentation appears to remove the main damaging factors in milk, our best dietary strategy is: *Switch from fluid milk to yogurt and cheese* (preferably in their low-fat and low-salt forms). However, it could be that in the diets of many people, the damaging factors in milk are not counterbalanced with enough of the protective foods (whole grains, vegetables and fruits).

There has been a strong emphasis in this country on the considerable need of women for calcium to avoid osteoporosis after menopause. Current recommendations of many nutritionists are for an intake of calcium greater than 800 mg. per day. The emphasis should rather be on how to get current levels of dietary calcium into the bones. Absorbed calcium can go astray — it can get laid down in soft tissue, around the joints, on top of atherosclerotic plaque in the arteries, in the kidneys, and in the heart.

The real problem is the body's proper utilization of calcium, which depends upon many other nutrients. Recent research shows that the trace element boron helps keep calcium in the bones. Vitamin C and trace elements zinc and manganese also help. Magnesium is also an important mineral for helping to get proper control of calcium in the body.

There are some excellent alternative sources of calcium. Green leafy vegetables are an excellent source of both calcium and magnesium. From Hispanic culture, there are tortillas and beans. From Oriental culture, there is tofu, which is soy bean curd treated with calcium.

Some additional vegetables that are good sources of calcium and magnesium are broccoli, cabbage, string beans, carrots, onions and tomatoes. Eggs and peas have adequate calcium. Oranges have good calcium, but it is mainly in the pulp, not in the juice. Meats, unfortunately, contain little calcium and are loaded with phosphorus, which hinders calcium absorption. Soft drinks have similar bad effects.

Primitive man must have sat around the campfire at night and chewed on bones — and no doubt those who grind their teeth in their sleep (bruxism) are trying to do that. Bruxism can often be cured with additional calcium and magnesium. Supplements of bone meal, oyster shell, or egg are good sources of calcium. Dolomite contains both calcium and magnesium in a good ratio between the two. However, because of a small (but real) risk of lead being in bonemeal or dolomite supplements, you might wish to use other calcium or magnesium sources. There are also various chelated calcium or magnesium supplements, which are better absorbed. One should take magnesium as well as calcium, never calcium alone. (Note an exception: People with kidney failure must usually avoid magnesium supplements, following the instructions of the physician.)

If you want to watch fat and salt, you might consider using part-skim or low-salt cheese. Mozzarella is a good example, but imitation cheeses are bad news nutritionally. It is uncertain whether or not cottage cheese or buttermilk escape the problems caused by fluid milk. Try to avoid most ice cream, loaded with milk and refined sugars.

The idea that yogurt promotes health and longevity is certainly not new. The low-fat type is preferred and it should contain a live culture; that is, it should not be pasteurized after being cultured. Plain yogurt, a bit too tart for most American tastes, will have listed about 125 calories per cup and 13 grams carbohydrate per cup. The heavily sweetened form is like a dessert and may have 250 calories per cup and 45 grams carbohydrate per cup. There is a happy medium somewhere in between.

For switching from milk to cheese or yogurt, you'll want to know the calcium equivalents: A cup of milk has roughly the same amount of calcium as a cup of yogurt, i.e., about 290 milligrams. Although cheeses vary considerably in calcium content, it takes about one and a third ounces of cheese to provide the calcium equivalent of a glass of milk.

It is helpful to remember that cow's milk is designed for baby cows — with super high protein and calcium to support the rapid growth rate of a calf — and needs modifying for human consumption.

Controlling Cholesterol

Some of the most nutritious foods are rich in cholesterol. It also happens to be a very natural material in our bodies, so it should not be feared. If you don't eat it, your body will produce more of it. Also remember that your body makes many vital substances from cholesterol.

In optimum health, cholesterol production is regulated so that blood serum cholesterol levels run 130 to 150 milligrams per deciliter. However, with blood cholesterol above about 240 mg/dl, the risk of heart disease is doubled. Above 300, the risk is tripled. The possibilities of lowering blood cholesterol levels by restricting dietary cholesterol are rather limited, with typical effects being blood cholesterol reductions of 5 to 15%. Frequently, the effect only lasts a matter of months, with blood cholesterol returning to the previous levels. This suggests that high blood cholesterol levels are a problem of the body's regulation of it, rather than of excessive dietary intake.

There is somewhat better luck lowering blood cholesterol levels (and stopping atherosclerosis) by going to completely vegetarian diets that are almost totally lacking in cholesterol. Most likely, such a diet is successful more because it is rich in nutrients and fiber than because it is low in dietary cholesterol. The additional nutrients probably make the body's cholesterol regulating mechanisms work better. With a rather strict diet, Nathan Pritikin drove his blood cholesterol down to 94 mg/dl — an abnormally low level. It had been 280 in the mid-1950's, before he changed his diet. He had been diagnosed as having "coronary insufficiency" from an electrocardiogram. However, upon autopsy after his death in 1985, he was found to have beautifully clean arteries. Most likely, there had been a reversal of atherosclerosis.

However, I doubt that one needs to go to such dietary extremes to have reasonably clean arteries; the right vitamin/mineral supplements can do as well. There are perhaps twenty different vitamins, minerals, or food factors that can lower blood cholesterol levels. The nutrients that can be effective are: vitamin A, vitamin C, niacin, vitamin B-6, choline, inositol, pangamate, essential fatty acid (especially omega-3 oil), and the minerals magnesium, calcium, copper, chromium, vanadium, nickel and silicon.

There seems to be a factor in yogurt that lowers blood cholesterol levels. Other effective food factors are apple pectin, oat bran, fresh raw carrot juice, and lecithin.

Drug approaches to lowering blood cholesterol levels have been plagued by side effects such as nausea, bloating, gas, or constipation. Results are better using the biochemical enabling action of nutrients to normalize cholesterol levels, rather than the biochemical blocking actions of drugs.

If your blood cholesterol level is elevated, improve your diet and try supplementing the nutrients that lower blood cholesterol. Then you can stop worrying about cholesterol.

Fear Of Fats

The conventional thinking on coronary heart disease has generated a neurotic fear of fats. Then how come total fat consumption has been rising steadily over the past century and a quarter?

There are several facts we need to help straighten out the confusion: We have an innate taste for fat and much of food fat is hidden. That is, we don't realize or want to know it is there. Food technologists find that processed foods containing fat sell well — thus they are more than willing to accommodate our tastes.

Relax, though. *Fat is not inherently bad.* The problem in a high fat diet is that the fats have displaced other foods of a higher nutrient-density. Health problems coming from a high fat diet most likely result from the lack of other protective nutrients that help your body handle fats.

Those Western countries with the highest total fat intake seem to have an excess of coronary heart disease over and above what one would expect from the dietary calcium to magnesium ratio. Fat calories were nearly a half of total calories. But how is it that the Masai, the Samburu, the Somali tribesmen, and the Tibetan nomads can get away with diets of about two-thirds fat calories and have virtually no heart disease? If any group of people can get away with such high fat consumption, then fat can not be a direct cause of coronary heart disease. Very likely, high fat is a contributor to coronary heart disease in Western countries because of other nutritional imbalances that disturb fat metabolism.

My guess is that the high dietary sodium to potassium ratio is one important imbalance, and another is probably the low dietary magnesium intake common in Western countries. Dietary refined grains and sugars adversely affect both factors.

Another problem of a high fat diet in Western countries is that the fats get modified or have other toxic substances inadvertently added and there is apt to be a hazard in vegetable oils processed in certain ways. Heating of polyunsaturated vegetable oils causes chemical changes, so some of the molecules will end up in an alien form. Also, the solvents used in processing cannot be completely removed.

If you insist on eating margarine, at least pick one, such as a tub margarine, that has a maximum of polyunsaturated oils and a minimum of hydrogenation which produces fats that cannot be utilized well by your body's cells. For myself, I prefer sweet (unsalted) butter and cold-pressed vegetable oils. Note that sweet butter should be stored in the freezer to prevent rancidity. Vegetable oils also turn rancid when stored for long periods of time.

For those who are weight conscious, note that fats give you nine Calories per gram, the highest of the three food categories. For comparison, proteins and carbohydrates only give you four Calories per gram. It is useful to know that removing 100 Calories per day from your food intake will cause you to lose about one pound per month, assuming your metabolism is normal. Of fatty foods, this is represented by one tablespoon of butter, oil, margarine, or mayonnaise. Two tablespoons of sugar, or 1 oz. of 100 proof liquor, would also have equivalent calories.

It is handy to know that it takes a much larger portion of vegetables to equal a fatty food in calories, since vegetables have a high water and fiber content. Be aware that a salad with an oil dressing on it is apt to have most of its calories in fat. Do not be deceived by regular ground beef advertised as 20% fat by weight, for it actually has two-thirds of its calories in fat. Many cheeses, including the very popular American process cheeses, are 70 to 75% fat calories. You may not realize the full extent of your fat consumption, since, like sugar and salt, much of it is hidden. Food manufacturers know that we have tastes for sugar, salt and fat and make full use of that to get us to buy their products.

Some extremists recommend a diet containing only 10% fat. With the right spices, such a diet can even be tasty. But in low-fat diets, problems may occur with absorption of fat soluble vitamins A, D, E and K, and with inadequate essential fatty acids. Diets as low as 20% fat can make cell membranes more rigid, blood plasma more viscous, and reduce immune system function.

The average American diet of 40 to 50% fat is likely too much, because of the many modified foods we eat. Consider the fact that high fat diets tend to promote cancer, especially of the colon and rectum. However, if you get substantial fiber in your diet, you will gain some protection. Supplementation with vitamins A, C and E will confer additional protection. Also, you must get some EPA (eicosapentaenoic acid), either from capsules or cold-water fish, for high fat diets block your body from making EPA from omega-3 oils. Thus, if you insist on having a high fat intake, take the necessary steps to protect yourself.

"Bad Habit" Scoreboard

There are important interactions — synergisms — between bad habits and nutritional factors (synergism being the interaction of two factors to generate a combined effect many times what was expected). In the combined effect of smoking and exposure to asbestos dust, for example, the risks of lung cancer are far greater than expected from either risk alone.

This same phenomenon of synergism is likely to occur between nutritional imbalances and so-called bad habits.

Let me cover the most common bad habits in turn: smoking, stress (type "A" behavior), drinking, lack of exercise (or excessive exercise), obesity, drugs, and violent behavior. The tendency to have accidents will also be considered.

Smoking

Among the benefits, smokers say that it helps energize them for work and that it reduces appetite, helping to control weight.

Among the risks, other than setting fires accidentally, are some very real health problems, such as lung cancer, emphysema, and heart disease. Statistical calculations suggest that Americans who smoke one pack per day have three times the risk of heart disease, and five times the combined risk of heart disease or cancer. But no valid conclusions can be drawn from the statistics because the influences of nutritional imbalances have not been taken into account. I would surmise that many who smoke are not particularly health conscious, and perhaps eat junk food as well. To believe any statistics on smoking risks, I would want to see data on smokers whose diets are close to optimum nutrition.

The world's heaviest smokers are in Greece, a country where there is a very low rate of coronary heart disease, and where the 45-year old male has a greater life expectancy than in any other country. Japanese and Chinese men are also extremely heavy smokers, and have low rates of coronary heart disease. In all these countries, the people eat food that is less sophisticated, less refined, closer to a primitive diet than what Americans eat. There is a good chance that optimum nutrition could drastically reduce the risks of continuing to smoke. Definitely, what you eat is more important than whether or not you smoke.

Stress Type "A" Behavior

In type "A" behavior, stress feeds upon itself and becomes reinforced over and over. Symptoms of this behavior are irritability, overactivity, intense drive, sense of urgency, hostility, inability to relax, worrying and insomnia.

Curiously, a number of stress symptoms are similar to those of magnesium depletion because stress depletes you of magnesium, and magnesium depletion enhances the bad effects of stress. Magnesium would seem to have a key role in preventing the body from overreacting to stresses.

Nutritional therapy can have an important role in preventing stress damage. Practically all nutrient needs are increased during stress. Vitamin C may be the most important nutrient lost during stress, but B-complex and magnesium run a close second. The all-American low-magnesium diet helps to make stress an important risk factor in coronary heart disease. With optimum nutrition and good vitamin and mineral supplementation, stress should not be a risk factor at all.

Drinking

There are some very important nutrient losses noted in heavy drinkers. Among them are vitamins A, C, E, B-1, B-6, B-12, niacin, folate and the minerals calcium, magnesium and zinc. (Iron may appear to be lost, according to blood measurements, but it tends to accumulate in the liver.) No doubt many other nutrients are lost as well, so that complete nutritional therapy for heavy drinkers would be a wise move.

Alcohol is addictive, and many who decide to quit will have difficulties quitting. Involved in alcohol addiction are genetic and psychological factors, as well as nutritional-biochemical factors. But before you decide to take up "religion" or long term psychotherapy to help you quit, note that there is an amino acid supplement, glutamine, that can help many quit without side effects. It takes about 2 grams of glutamine per day (500 mg doses at each meal and at bedtime) to do the job. Glutamine can be obtained from your local health food store or from mail-order vitamin companies.

Lack of Exercise — Excessive Exercise

In our society, we have a tendency to confuse fitness with health. No amount of physical training can guarantee you a healthy heart. You can appear to be (and feel) physically fit, but you might still be on the verge of a heart attack. Optimum nutrition gives you the best chance of having a healthy heart. In fact, if you are not getting optimum nutrition, it is best to avoid heavy exercise.

Moderate exercise does have some benefits — it increases HDL, the good lipoprotein in the blood. Exercise helps keep calcium in your bones. It also helps burn off calories that might otherwise go into fat. One advantage of a nutritional therapy program is that it will make you feel more like exercising.

You should be aware of certain physiological effects of exercise on your body. Exercise causes release of endorphins, which are sort of a natural "morphine." Thus exercise is likely to make you feel better. The danger is that exercise can easily be overdone, resulting in injuries. Also, note that excess exercise, such as running more than 40 miles per week, has been shown to lower testosterone levels and sex drive.

Obesity

It is true that obesity results from too high a caloric intake relative to the exercise level, but other problems could also be present. The metabolism may have gone awry, so that the individual is unable to burn fuel fast enough or the appetite mechanism may not be functioning well. Since these problems are at the cellular level, there is a reasonable chance that getting all the essential nutrients to the cells may correct the problem.

Forget about all those heavily advertised "crash" diets. They will foul up your metabolism in such a way you will actually *gain* weight in the long run. The only effective long-term diet is moderate calorie restriction, especially of foods that have many calories and few nutrients, such as sugar, fats, oils and alcohol. Add to this an increased exercise level, plus vitamin and mineral supplements.

There is some evidence that adding omega-3 oil to the diet will increase your body's heat production so that you'll burn off more fat. For these purposes, the best source of omega-3 oil is food-grade linseed oil. Of course, you must remove enough other fats and oils from your diet to compensate for the added calories of the linseed oil.

It has recently been found that artificial sweeteners won't help you lose weight. The evidence is that they whet your appetite so you will eat other foods that contain calories. Also, the more fat in your diet, the more calories you'll tend to consume, and the more weight you'll gain. Thus, dietary fat whets your appetite for more food.

Drugs

There are many ways of categorizing drugs: as legal or illegal, prescription or over-the-counter, socially acceptable or not, addictive or not, stimulants or tranquillizers (uppers or downers), safe or dangerous, psychoactive or not, etc.

Alcohol, coffee and tea have to be included as drugs. Note that the caffeine in coffee or tea can have some benefits, but three or more cups per day of coffee can cause a significant loss of nutrients from your body.

An important aspect of drugs is that they tend to have anti-nutrient effects. Aspirin will deplete you of vitamin C and folic acid, barbiturates interfere with vitamin D metabolism, diuretics will knock out B-complex and C vitamins, plus calcium, magnesium, potassium, and zinc; and Digitalis tends to knock out vitamin B-1, magnesium, and potassium.

The body builds up tolerance to increasing doses of many drugs, and nutritional therapies can be helpful in getting off addictive drugs but have been little publicized.

The best news is that vitamin C in large doses can be immensely helpful when you are trying to quit an addictive drug cold-turkey. In order to avoid bloating your belly with large doses, it must be oral dosages of a non-acidic form of vitamin C, such as calcium ascorbate or sodium ascorbate. 1 to 2 grams *per hour*, are considered reasonable for kicking heavy drugs like heroin. If you can find a knowledgeable physician or clinic that helps people quit, you can get vitamin C intravenously. Kicking milder drugs like coffee may require only a few grams per day of vitamin C.

The urge to do drugs, the risks of addiction, and the risks of a bad trip are probably all increased when an individual is in a poor nutritional state. With the aid of nutritional therapy, people can kick a habit more comfortably. The withdrawal blues can be reduced using vitamins with the amino acid tyrosine.

Violence

How do we interpret the fact that the consumption of several foods — meat, milk or sugar — correlates statistically to violence? Meat seems to increase aggressiveness in men. Milk may contribute to hyperexcitability through its high calcium to magnesium ratio, or by triggering a cerebral allergy. Typical amounts of sugar consumption in the U. S. A. can lead to hypoglycemia, which is a fertile source of antisocial behavior. It was found that 90% of the men in one jail were hypoglycemic. By shifting diets toward foods having a higher nutrient-density (avoiding sugars, excessive fat, and food additives), various juvenile detention facilities have experienced substantial decreases in antisocial behavior among inmates.

An excess of copper can lead to a proneness to violence. Accumulation of toxic metals like lead may contribute to hyperexcitability and violence in some people. Alcohol and drug habits have been suggested as causing much violence. However, the more fundamental problem may be the poor nutritional state of people on alcohol, on drugs, or with accumulated lead.

It would be a mistake to try to ascribe any "main causes" to violence. There are a variety of contributing factors that interact and develop over a long period of time. A poor diet may act like a trigger and destroy an individual's chances of bettering his life. Thus, in an adverse social milieu, he might find that the easiest path to take is one leading to crime and violence.

Accidents

Hypoglycemia could put you into a state of mind where you become accident prone. If you are deficient in zinc and/or copper, you may get a tendency to "space out" a bit. That can contribute to an accident. If you are in a marginal nutritional state relative to zinc, switching to a vegetarian diet (normally healthy) could give you a "spacy" feeling.

A non-nutritional factor is the depletion of negative air ions. The modern design of our cities, our buildings and our cars have a tendency to knock them out. Places where you'll find a rich supply of negative ions are at the seashore, next to waterfalls, in the shower and in the woods on a breezy day. If such places make you feel a lot better, you might also want to try out a negative ion generator in your home, office or car.

If the air is well charged with negative ions, you are apt to feel good, but if it is charged with positive ions (or none) then accident rates go up and heart attacks are more frequent.

Keeping Your Head Straight

When people are hurting in the mind, their best strategy might be to see a nutritional therapist. If the root of the problem is inadequate nutrition, no amount of psychotherapy will cure it. Even if the primary root of the problem is in the psychologic realm, nutritional therapy can probably help shorten the period of psychotherapy needed.

Your mental well-being depends upon genetic, nutritional and environmental factors. Additionally, the attitudes you choose to take toward your life situation are extremely important. Thus it looks as if there is free will. Even with free will, though, there is a chemical basis to your thought processes, the same as with other body processes. A less than optimum nutrition can adversely influence brain chemistry, and therefore interfere with normal thought processes. Studies, for example, have related depression to marginal deficiencies of vitamins B-1, B-2, B-6, B-12 or C. Deficiencies of, or an extra need for, any one of these vitamins can cause depression. Psychological symptoms almost always develop before any physical symptoms of the deficiency.

Consider some examples of nutrients that have been found to work in individual cases:

1. If you are a burn-out case, and have lost all your ambition, you might find a dramatic restoration of ambition by taking a few hundred milligrams per day of pantothenic acid.

2. If you are primarily involved in intellectual work, you may find that zinc and copper supplementation sharpens up your brain, allowing better creative imagination.

3. If you do physical work, you may find that iron supplements give you more energy to get the job done.

4. If you are a lethargic type of person, you may find that copper or bioflavonoids energize you.

5. If you are hyperactive (usually a male problem), driving everyone around you crazy, you may find that you have excess copper, or toxic levels of lead, or are getting too little magnesium for the amount of calcium, or have a food allergy.

6. If you are anxious much of the time or have insomnia, you may need more magnesium. Other cases of insomnia could be helped by GTF-chromium or by the amino acid tryptophan.

7. If you are irritable or have a bad temper, you might find great help from magnesium or GTF-chromium.

8. If your memory has been failing in recent years, you might need extra zinc and vitamin B-6 (especially if you have white spots on your fingernails), or magnesium, or choline.

9. If you need tranquilizing, you might find the answer in magnesium, zinc, inositol, vitamin C or vitamin E. On the other hand, if you take a prescription drug to calm yourself, you may become addicted to it.

10. If you get depressed too often, you might find relief with magnesium, GTF-chromium, B-complex and C vitamins, or amino acids phenylalanine or tyrosine.

Experimentation is necessary to find out what answers your own personal needs. Psychosocial factors need to be considered.

Also, any of the problems mentioned above could have its roots in a food allergy.

Sex And Nutrition

(Because this section is written from a male point of view, some women may not wish to read it. However, it has much useful information for women.)

We live in a youth oriented culture, but we obviously can't stay young forever. To maintain our attractiveness, we have to stave off the ravages of time. If you allow yourself to become fat, toothless and flatulent as you age, you will have to scale down your expectations. Also unattractive are a paunch, bags under the eyes, heavy body odors, prostate problems, heavy snoring, and feeling fatigued much of the time.

Many of the problems that interfere with your sexual attractiveness can be prevented, or even reversed, with optimum nutrition and nutritional therapy. No matter how far gone you are now, it is worth an effort. It will help you feel better about yourself and help keep a mate from deciding you are over the hill.

The male hormone testosterone is certainly a key to male sex drive. Super-aggressive males perhaps have too much of it being produced and floating around their system. Very passive men with minimal sex drive may be underproducing. If you are a regular marijuana smoker or a heavy drinker, you may find that your testosterone levels are low. The food preservative nitrate also lowers sex drive. Supplements of the amino-acid tyrosine may help low sex drive.

There are some nutrients that can influence sexual capabilities. They aren't likely to fulfill male fantasies of superhuman sexual feats, but they certainly can bring males up to normal — which is sexy enough. It is doubtful that young males need anything, although optimum nutrition raises the possibility of first-rate sexual performance without a dragged-out or spacy feeling the next day. You see, when you indulge heavily in sex, you use up nutrients and other biochemical compounds (enzymes) that are needed for other physical and mental functions.

One of the more important nutrients spent during sex is zinc. Each male orgasm causes the loss of one to two milligrams of zinc. That may require 5-10 milligrams in the diet to replace because zinc absorption in the gut is far below 100%. If you don't replace the zinc, you'll gradually deplete your body stores. Then, as you age, you may get a variety of ailments, including poorer intellectual functioning and prostate problems. Tiny white spots on your fingernails are one sure sign of zinc depletion.

One biochemical compound, histamine, is released during sexual arousal and leads to a blushing reaction and the warm feeling before orgasm. Men or women who are slow in or have difficulty achieving orgasm may need extra chemical precursors to histamine. One of the B-vitamins, folic acid, can serve this purpose well. Many will find benefit in taking folic acid tablets with their B-complex tablets.

Another nutrient, niacin (a form of vitamin B-3) is a precursor to histamine. Niacin is likely to elicit a positive response in 10 minutes, whereas the folic acid benefits happen in a matter of days and seem more natural. Even modest doses of niacin lead to a rapid flush reaction in most people, which is why B-complex tablets usually contain another form of the vitamin, niacinamide, which gets a slower response. You have to experiment to see what works best for you, but don't go overboard on any one nutrient, since that can create imbalances that disturb other biochemical functions.

The inability to get an erection may have psychological roots. It can also be physiological in nature. It is generally worth trying nutritional therapy first, since that can help reduce time needed for psychotherapy later. A gradual degeneration of the circulatory system with aging can lead to the loss of the ability to get an erection. That can be reversed partially by nutritional therapy. For a quick, temporary fix, a urologist can give you a local injection of a vasodilator drug.

Now let us look into what can be done to improve your sexual attractiveness. Nutritional therapy, tailored to the individual, can frequently do wonders, but may take many months to work.

Obesity

The important steps to weight reduction are cutting down on calorie intake, switching to foods of higher nutrient density, increasing exercise, and fixing up a faulty appetite mechanism (or faulty metabolism) by using vitamin and mineral supplements. Also, sex is excellent exercise. In other words, take your mate rather than a plate.

Having a paunch

Although genetic factors are apt to be important, you can improve matters by exercising the belly muscles. For keeping your connective tissues from failing and letting your innards sag, the most important nutrients are vitamins C and B-6, copper and silicon. The same applies to sagging jowls and neck wattles.

Bags under the eyes

This is a sign of excess fluid in the tissues. However, if you have dark circles around the eyes, you may have allergies, or be getting too little sleep. To drive out fluid and tighten tissues, the most important nutrients are vitamins C and B-6, copper and silicon. Nutritional therapy can do almost as well as a face lift but may require a year's time to notice a difference.

Flatulence

This means excessive gas, either trapped and causing you pain or released with social embarrassment. Too many legumes (dry beans, soy beans or lentils) or improperly prepared legumes can do it. People with lactose intolerance get gas from milk and its products, except from aged cheese. Some people may need yogurt and more food fiber regularly to keep the right bacteria working in the lower intestine. Food allergies also cause gas. Or you may be producing too little stomach acid or pancreatic juices, which can often be corrected through nutritional therapy.

Heavy body odors

Deficiencies of either magnesium or zinc can contribute to excessive odors. Deodorants and antiperspirants work partly by blocking your skin pores. They don't get at the real, biochemical problem.

Heavy snoring

If your snoring is as loud as a 747 taking off, or a jackhammer at 10 feet, you probably have a health problem (and your partner has a sleeping problem). I know that there are some nutrients that help, for I was a heavy snorer before trying vitamins and minerals but a fairly light one afterwards. Heavy snoring is a risk factor for coronary heart disease.

Hair loss with aging

Heredity appears to be one of the more important factors here, but it is possible to slow down the loss with optimum nutrition. The shortage of (or extra need for) almost any nutrient can contribute to premature hair loss, but zinc and high quality protein are perhaps the most important factors. After trying vitamins and minerals for a few months, some people find a profuse number of new hairs growing just outside the hairline. Receding of the hairline appears to slow down as long as the supplements are continued.

Prostate problems

Usually these involve enlargement, bacterial infection or cancer. The bladder is pushed aside by the enlarged prostate, so that bladder capacity is reduced, and one has to get up during the night to urinate. Zinc is the most protective nutrient for the prostate gland, but essential fatty acids, vitamin E, vitamin A and vitamin B-6 help get zinc back into the gland. Many men have had prostate enlargement disappear using these supplements, and thus have avoided the surgical knife. Since it takes a year to get the results, and unfortunately doesn't seem to work with all men, prevention is best.

Hemorrhoids

Essentially, these are varicose veins of the anus. From the commercials with the evening TV news, you may gather that there is big money in preparations to relieve hemorrhoid symptoms. You can bet that they don't advertise in the less developed countries, since hemorrhoids don't tend to exist there. About one out of three Americans suffers from hemorrhoids. While stress can make latent hemorrhoids act up, it is certainly not the cause. The problem is one of nutrition and is cured by adding extra fiber, vitamins A, C, E and B-6, essential fatty acids and bioflavonoids. The fiber helps bring the fecal cylinder up to normal size (larger) so that the evacuation mechanisms can work easily without straining at stool. You should increase fiber gradually, to avoid getting a blockage. The nutrients help restore the structures and restart the glands that produce the lubricants that aid stool passage. Once you get your defecation equipment working right, you'll find that you spend only a minute on the throne, that it is a pleasant experience, and that there is little or no soilage around the anus.

Frequent illnesses

If you get illnesses more than a few times per year, optimum nutrition can strengthen your immune system. It needs all the essential nutrients for proper functioning, but the nutrients that appear most important are folic acid, zinc, and vitamins B-6, B-12, C, and omega-3 oil. Also helpful are bioflavonoids and pangamate. Vitamin A can help you resist bacterial infections, while lysine can help resist viral attacks. Note that stress can make your immune system work less well, but with optimum nutrition, stress may be unimportant. Too many polyunsaturated oils in your diet, or high doses of vitamin E (1000 i.u.) can also impair normal immune system functioning.

For those whose immune systems are hypersensitive, i.e., they get allergies, a high dose of vitamin E and less dietary protein may be the answer.   Identifying allergies and eliminating the problem substances will give your immune system a better chance of fighting off the real enemies (bacteria and viruses).

When your body is responding to infection with a fever, supplementation may not be wise, so fortify your system while you are well.

Of course, you don't need to get rid of these health problems just for sexual reasons.   You'll find a greater overall enjoyment of life in many ways.

Assorted Hazards

Hardly a day goes by that the newspapers or TV aren't exposing a new environmental hazard − pollution of our air, food, drinking water, workplace, or even our homes, with toxic metals, pesticide residues, defoliants, herbicides, solvents and other exotic chemicals.   There is an excellent way of protecting ourselves from these dangers and that is by enhancing our own body's natural defenses with optimum nutrition and with certain supplements.

Among the assorted hazards are the *free radicals*, which are high-energy fragments of molecules, produced in our bodies by low-level radiation, toxins, rancid oils and even as a side effect of normal metabolic processes.   Free radicals create havoc by attacking the structures of the body's cells and interfering in normal biochemical processes.   The anti-oxidant nutrients − vitamins A, C, and E and the mineral selenium − work at destroying free radicals before they can do damage.

Pesticides, exotic chemicals and solvents have found their way into the water table in many parts of the country so a good spring water is perhaps healthiest.

For general protection against environmental pollutants, wherever they are found, you can take daily supplements of vitamins A, C and E. The appropriate dosages for most people are in the range of 10,000 to 25,000 i.u. of vitamin A, 1,000 to 4,000 mg of vitamin C, and 100 to 400 i.u. of vitamin E. Note that the U.S. RDA's take no account of the extra need for nutrients because of environmental pollutants. You've probably heard "experts" warning you against vitamin A dosage at these levels, but they never seem to tell you that vitamin E will protect you from vitamin A overdosage. Note well that once you've been on supplementation of vitamins C and E for awhile, you should not abruptly quit supplementation, for that will bring on deficiency symptoms. If you plan to quit, then taper off the dosage over several months' time.

We are all being exposed to *toxic metals*, some more so than others. In dealing with the toxic metals — lead, aluminum, cadmium, mercury and arsenic — fortifying your own body's defenses is all-important.

Lead

A number of nutrients will help prevent lead absorption or help clear it from the body. It is most important to get adequate amounts of the minerals calcium, magnesium, zinc, iron and selenium. Vitamins C and E are important. Methionine, an essential amino acid that is rich in eggs, helps clear lead. Lactose (milk sugar) promotes lead absorption.

Aluminum

A generous magnesium intake does the best job of blocking aluminum absorption. Phosphate and fluoride also work against the absorption of the 50 milligrams or so of aluminum that goes through your gut every day. Antacids that contain aluminum hydroxide are best avoided. It is not wise to cook or store acidic foods (citrus, tomato, cherry or rhubarb) or oxalate foods (spinach, other greens) in aluminum pots. In the brain, aluminum leads to an early and irreversible senility.

Cadmium

When cadmium is absorbed by your body, it tends to accumulate in the outer layers of the kidney and lead to high blood pressure. You can help your body block cadmium absorption by getting adequate zinc and selenium. Some other nutrients that also help are calcium, copper, iron and vitamin C.

Mercury

Mercury compounds can poison the brain. Its sources are some fungicides used on grain seeds, or fish from waters downstream from industrial plants that make paper pulp or chlorine. Dentists are much at risk from breathing in mercury vapors while making mercury fillings. About 1% of people are hypersensitive, and can't take mercury fillings in the mouth. While selenium supplementation may be helpful in preventing problems with mercury, it can't do much about curing mercury poisoning.

Arsenic

A little bit of arsenic is good for you; in fact, it is an essential nutrient. However, too much will do you in. Getting adequate selenium is the best protection from excessive arsenic.

In summary, your best strategy against all the environmental hazards is to:

1. Mobilize your own body's natural defenses with optimum nutrition and the specific supplements that help.
2. Avoid the worst of the hazards around you.
3. Then quit worrying.

Enjoyment Of Food

We have to keep in mind that foods are for enjoyment as well as for nutrition and health. Every culture develops its own food habits, and these habits evolve with time. Those cultures that maintain a strong tradition of nutritious foods and eating habits can flourish for the longest time with their peoples in the best health. However, in the U. S. A., we seem to be developing a melting-pot cuisine of foods that are smooth, require a minimum of chewing, and can be bolted down fast. The foods are devoid of fiber and loaded with sugar, salt and fat. When combined with two major staples like refined flour and milk, the result is a high rate of male heart disease.

A health-protective diet can also be an enjoyable diet. We don't really need most of the products of modern food technology. After you get used to whole foods, your taste buds will change. Thus the old-fashioned foods will seem tastier than the modern ones. You'll find that white bread tastes like cardboard, and you'll recognize when someone has laced your food with sugar or salt. Some of your old favorites are likely to taste too greasy. It will be a whole new world of food for you to explore with your "normalized" taste buds.

Using the concepts of nutrient-density, we can develop a far better ranking of foods. The foods with the highest nutrient-density are the most health-protective foods, in almost all cases. They have the most nutrients, or broadest spectrum of nutrients for the amount of calories.

The *first* rank on this scale would be certain vegetables and liver. These are almost complete in all nutrients. Some examples of vegetables with the highest nutrient-density are string beans, carrots, peas, cabbage, spinach, lettuce, or other fleshy or leafy vegetables. Strange as it may seem, liver is first rank, for it is lacking in only one nutrient, calcium. A few pounds of liver will give you a whole day's supply of calories. However, liver has too much vitamin A, so you shouldn't have a serving of it more than twice per week.

In *second* rank would be all the sources of high-grade animal protein: meat, fowl, fish, oysters, eggs and certain milk products. Men should only take fluid milk in their coffee or tea. Fermented milks, such as yogurt or kefir, are excellent. Strangely, when milk is converted to cheese, it loses much nutrient-density but becomes a protective food for men. For vegetarians, legumes (dry beans, lentils and soybeans) combined with the right grains can provide reasonable protein.

Third rank would be whole grains, which are the best source of fiber and an important source of starch, along with vegetables like potatoes. Get variety in grains, selecting from wheat, rye, brown rice, corn, barley, oats, buckwheat, millet, etc.

Fourth rank would be fruits, which are a main source of vitamin C. (Vitamin C tends to get cooked out of other foods.) They are also a good source of bioflavonoids and certain useful fibers. But fruit fibers don't give much "bulking" action compared to grain fibers.

The *fifth* rank would be essential oils (polyunsaturates) from sources such as avocados, nuts, fish, peanut butter, mayonnaise, or extracted seed oils. Only a modest amount of oil is needed per day.

Most people get too much oil and not the right kind. You need more sources of omega-3 oil, both from vegetables sources (oils from linseed, walnut, wheat germ or soy) and fish sources (cold-water fish containing eicosapentaenoic acid, EPA, and docosahexaenoic acid, DHA). If you have a high-fat diet (like the majority of Americans), and don't eat much fish, it is wise to take EPA/"fish oil" capsules. The easiest way to get your omega-3 oil is from food-grade linseed oil, available from health food stores (not hardware stores) and the best oil is extracted mechanically at cold temperatures. The average person's requirement will be about one teaspoon per day.

If you get a combination of these five ranks, you'll cover all nutrients in generous amounts. The more of the four highest rank foods you get, the more protection you get against illness and disease. Note that for men, milk must take a very low rank, because of its special problems, previously discussed. Your calcium will come from cheese, yogurt, dark green leafy vegetables or certain ethnic foods like tofu or tortillas. Also note that wilted, overcooked, canned or frozen vegetables have to go into a lower ranking than fresh ones.

There is another rank, which I'll call *bottom* rank. Mostly, they are the refined, partitioned, fractured or manufactured foods. You may eat modestly from this category, but only as a calculated risk. Nothing will happen to you right away, or for years, but over decades they may take a toll. The category includes most fats and oils, refined grains (white flour, white rice, degerminated corn meal), sugar, salt and alcohol. Most ice creams, combining milk and sugar, are on the restricted list, especially for men.

Descending further, nutritionally speaking, we have wine and hard liquor. Wine is replete with natural toxins left over from the fermentation, plus dozens of man-made additives allowed by law but not listed on any labels. Hard liquor has zero nutrient-density, but at least charcoal filtering may have taken out some toxic substances. The main toxin remaining is ethyl alcohol. Only vodka and beer appear to be free of urethane, a carcinogen.

Besides food rank or nutrient-density, there are other considerations. Variety in foods is important. Anyone who restricts himself to just a few foods, even the best of foods, or skips any of the top five ranks, is setting himself up for possible problems, either from deficiencies or from natural food toxins. At the other extreme, too much variety also carries a risk, since your taste buds may get overstimulated and lead you to overeat and put on weight.

Most people feel better and have more energy when they are getting some of the high-grade protein foods from animal sources: meat, fish, fowl, eggs, cheese or yogurt. But those who get too many of the animal protein foods, with too few of the other protective foods, may be setting themselves up for trouble. Vegetables provide important protective nutrients.

The time of day you eat food can make a difference. If you tend to eat mainly one large meal per day in the evening, you may find a tendency to gain weight. Those who skip breakfast, or just do a coffee and donut routine, are apt to find their energy flagging during the day. If that is happening to you, try eating a high-protein breakfast, and then concentrate more on the protective foods for the rest of the day. You may be better able to experience all-day energy this way.

My recommendation on diets is: don't wait for that magic new diet that will come out next week — just stick to the high nutrient-density foods, cut down on your total calories, get more exercise and take vitamin and mineral supplements. You have to experiment to find what works best for you. Once you discover the best foods for yourself, you have won at least half the battle.

Proper Use Of Supplements

It is wise to remember that the physical symptoms of a health problem arrive in a late stage of a nutritional deficiency. The earlier stages include depletion of body stores, then biochemical abnormalities, followed by mental symptoms. An excellent argument for supplements is that they may allow you to get away with a bad habit or two with less risk, so let us cover in greater detail the individual nutrients, including some of their interactions.

The Vitamins

Vitamin A

Vitamin A is best known for preventing night blindness, but it is important to the health of all tissues, especially the skin and various mucous linings of the body. It is also helpful as cancer protection. You have to experiment to find your own optimum vitamin A dose, but it will probably range from 10,000 to 50,000 i.u. daily.

B-complex Vitamins

You'll find B-complex tablets in dosages from RDA amounts (a few milligrams each of B-1, 2, 6, with a few micrograms of B-12) up to 150 milligrams of each. The better quality tablets will have as much B-6 as B-1, and tend to include up to 11 different B-complex factors.

Most characteristically, the B-complex factors help in nerve or nervous disorders, but can also help in a hundred other problems. We'll examine the individual B-complex factors.

Thiamine (B-1)

Inadequate amounts of thiamine can lead to low energy, or to beri-beri. Alcohol, drugs, stress and many other factors can deplete you of thiamine. If you have a magnesium deficiency, it may manifest itself as a seemingly high need for thiamine.

Riboflavin (B-2)

Most of the problems found with a riboflavin deficiency are not especially unique to a riboflavin deficiency. But if you get cracks and sores in the corners of the mouth, a red sore tongue, or dry burning eyes, you might try riboflavin supplementation first. Riboflavin deficiency also contributes to eye cataracts. Alcohol, drugs, stress and other factors can deplete you of riboflavin.

Niacin, niacinamide (B-3)

The RDA for niacin is 18 milligrams. Typical B-complex tablets have 100 mg. of the niacinamide form of B-3. The niacinamide form is generally used in supplements, since 100 mg. of the niacin form can cause a skin flush reaction, which could be alarming to someone who doesn't expect it.

Pantothenic acid (B-5)

The National Academy of Sciences says that the "safe and adequate" dose of pantothenic acid is 4 to 7 mg. daily. However, I've never heard of any problems with taking thousands of milligrams daily. But start with 100 mg., and work up, finding the level which works best for you. It's certainly a useful vitamin against stress, allergy and aging. It can help some individuals recover lost ambition. Refined foods cheat you of pantothenic acid.

Pyridoxine (B-6)

The RDA for vitamin B-6 is 2.2 mg. But don't limit yourself to that amount unless you want minimum health. It's my guess that about 10% of the population have a vitamin *B-6 dependency*, needing amounts they could never get from food in order to maintain optimum health.

Vitamin B-6 can sometimes fix up a failing memory. Your ability to recall your dreams when you wake up gives a good measure of your short-term memory.

Vitamin B-6 can also help prevent atherosclerosis. An adequate dosage for this purpose is perhaps 25 to 50 mg. per day.

Almost always, you should supplement magnesium along with vitamin B-6. If you don't, you may find yourself getting irritable and having insomnia.

There is an important interaction between vitamin B-6 and omega-3 oil. If you have a vitamin B-6 dependency, you may find that it seems to disappear after you get a rich source of omega-3, such as linseed oil, one teaspoon daily for a month.

Cobalamin (B-12)

Since vitamin B-12 is found almost exclusively in animal products, strict vegetarians may have trouble getting enough B-12. The RDA is 3 micrograms (0.003 milligrams). Unfortunately, some people develop a vitamin B-12 dependency which may come on insidiously with aging. The body's inability to utilize B-12 can lead to inadequate stomach acid being produced, pernicious anemia, or mental problems. In such cases, even large oral doses can not be adequately absorbed, so that vitamin B-12 injections are needed.

Biotin

Between dietary sources (liver and other high protein foods) and production by your intestinal bacteria, most people get adequate biotin (100 to 200 micrograms). Biotin deficiency can cause many different health problems. Taking antibiotics can cause a biotin deficiency, but the intestinal flora can be restored by taking some yogurt. If you are in the habit of eating raw egg whites, you are likely headed for trouble, for a protein in raw eggs will bind up biotin. The higher quality B-complex tablets contain some biotin.

Folic acid

High-powered B-complex tablets are relatively short on folic acid, for no tablet is allowed to contain more than 0.4 mg. (400 micrograms). Thus extra folic acid tablets may be appropriate in order to achieve a better balance of the B-complex factors. The restriction on folic acid in vitamin supplements in the U. S. A. is intended to help doctors recognize cases of pernicious anemia. If you have signs such as anemia, poor appetite, considerable weight loss, vague abdominal pains, burning tongue, or even temporary loss of sensations in the extremities, you should get checked out by a physician for the possibility of pernicious anemia, *before* you start taking folic acid supplements.

Choline

The better quality B-complex tablets will contain some choline, typically 250 mg. of choline bitartrate. Choline is needed all over the body, but nowhere more than in your nerve fibers, where it helps form the sheaths covering the fibers. It is also transformed into an important neurotransmitter substance, acetylcholine, which aids transfer of nerve impulses both to other nerve cells and to muscles. Choline can help rescue some people from early senility or failing memory.

Inositol

The richest source of both choline and inositol is lecithin, which is helpful to some people with elevated blood cholesterol or triglycerides, or with heart disease. If you take lecithin, be aware that it is loaded with phosphorus, and will thus increase your need for calcium and magnesium supplementation. B-complex tablets with choline will usually include an equal amount of inositol. Separate inositol tablets may be useful to some people who need tranquillizing or have insomnia. Other nutrients that could be helpful in such problems are magnesium, chromium, or tryptophan.

Para-aminobenzoic Acid

PABA for short. Your body can convert PABA to folic acid if your diet is deficient in folic acid, and thus spare you from anemia. It is included in the better B-complex tablets in 30 to 50 mg. amounts. PABA is often used externally, especially in sun-screen lotions.

Vitamin C

The RDA amount of vitamin C, 60 mg., would appear to be intended to achieve minimum health. Under stress, you need far more than 60 mg. of vitamin C. Many men will find their optimum dose around 2,000 mg. An excess of vitamin C will give you temporary diarrhea, but that usually requires a dose of about 5,000 mg. While some experiments haven't shown the efficacy of sizable doses of vitamin C in preventing the common cold, experiments on men under heavy stress (such as soldiers out on bivouac) have shown highly significant results.

I must warn you that, after you have been on long-term vitamin C supplementation, you should not stop taking it, for you may get deficiency symptoms. If you are planning to reduce vitamin C supplementation, taper off in your dosage over a period of a few months.

Vitamin C interacts with other nutrients. It promotes the absorption of iron, and interferes with copper. Because the all-American diet is short on copper, it would not be wise to take only vitamin C with such a diet.

Vitamin C has many different functions in maintaining human health. It is only man, the apes, monkeys and guinea pigs that are unable to produce vitamin C. All the other animals produce a quantity of vitamin C that is proportional to the amount of stress the animal is under.

Some experts warn about the possibility of kidney stones if you take large doses of vitamin C. However, kidney stones are only a possibility in about 1% of people and could easily be prevented by supplements of magnesium and vitamin B-6. If taking large doses, get a non-acidic form of vitamin C, such as calcium ascorbate or sodium ascorbate, to prevent stomach upsets. If diarrhea occurs, the dose should be cut back a bit. High doses (30 to 40 grams per day) appear appropriate for quitting heavy drug habits or to improve cancer survival.

Vitamin D

The RDA for adults is 200 i.u. If you are getting plenty of sunshine, there is no reason at all to get a vitamin D supplement. The sunshine in northern latitudes is adequate for whites, but not for blacks. Blacks living in northern latitudes should make sure that they get some vitamin D.

Because atmospheric pollutants like the chlorofluorocarbons (CFC) have been decreasing the ozone layer in the upper atmosphere, we now have a greater exposure to ultraviolet radiation. That has contributed to skin cancer rates going up and more rapid skin aging in people who get much sunshine. The use of sun-blocking lotions is reasonable prevention. However, if you are practicing optimum nutrition, you needn't be quite so paranoid about sunshine.

Vitamin E

Typical American diets have been found to contain from 8 to 24 i.u. of *d-alpha tocopherol*, which is the most biologically active form of vitamin E. There are also other forms of vitamin E in food: beta, gamma and delta tocopherol. The delta form is the least biologically active, but has the best anti-oxidant properties. Antioxidants are important for your body, for they keep oils from turning rancid and protect your body's cells from free radicals. The best anti-oxidant nutrients are vitamin C and E and selenium. As a supplement, the best form of vitamin E is either the d-alpha form or the mixed form, containing alpha, beta, gamma, delta and some rarer types.

Some foods lose most of their vitamin E during processing. Refined grains have lost almost all of their vitamin E, and frozen foods most of it. Overcooking or long storage will add to the losses. Oxygen is an enemy of vitamin E, either in food or in the body.

In the early space flights, the men ate freeze-dried foods and were breathing almost pure oxygen. During a flight, they lost about 25% of their red blood cells, becoming anemic, weakened and easily fatigued. On later flights, the food was supplemented with vitamin E, protecting the men. In a lack of sufficient vitamin E, particularly when breathing pure oxygen, all of the body's cell membranes are attacked by rancid oils and free radicals. Red blood cell membranes get weak and burst, and muscles start wasting.

Recent evidence shows that runners tend to become anemic, but cyclists don't. It appears that the pounding of the feet on the ground breaks red blood cells. There is no better way of protecting your red blood cells than by getting more whole foods and taking vitamin E supplements.

What sort of diet will give you the most vitamin E? Richest in vitamin E are freshly-ground whole grains and sweet potatoes. Nuts, freshly shelled, are rich in E. Eggs are adequate, but meat has insufficient E (on a calorie basis). Milk is totally lacking. If you have much meat or milk, you actually need additional vitamin E to protect the sulfur amino acids, such as methionine. If your diet is rich in polyunsaturated oils, you need more vitamin E.

With the seeming impossibility of getting the ideal diet, and with air and water pollution increasing vitamin E needs, I recommend vitamin E supplementation. An insurance dose would be 100 i.u. of the natural form. If you get no adverse side effects, a 400 i.u. capsule would be reasonable, especially in older people. As with vitamin C, you must not stop your vitamin E supplementation suddenly, or you are apt to get deficiency symptoms. The RDA, roughly 11 i.u., only insures minimum health.

Vitamin E protects from all manner of problems of the circulatory system — short-lived red blood cells, excessive tendency of the blood to clot, varicose veins, hemorrhoids, intermittent claudication (pains in the legs while walking, due to muscles starved of oxygen because of narrowed arteries), atherosclerosis, angina pectora (chest pains from oxygen-starved heart muscle), and coronary heart disease.

Vitamin E can also be useful externally, applied to burns, sunburn, rashes, and leg ulcers. It decreases pain and aids healing.

Essential Fatty Acids (EFA)

Some call this vitamin F. It includes certain polyunsaturated fatty acids: alpha-*linoleic* acid, an omega-6 oil and alpha-*linolenic* acid, an omega-3 oil. These are the basic building blocks of many substances your body needs, including all cell membranes, much of your brain, and the hormone-like prostaglandins. The richest food sources of linoleic are the most commonly used oils: safflower, corn, sunflower, cottonseed, and peanut. For linolenic, linseed oil is far and away the richest source, but oils like walnut, wheat germ, and soybean are reasonable sources. One teaspoon of food grade linseed oil per day can supply the need for omega-3.

There are many possible disorders if you get too little omega-3 oil, but the problems are not specific to omega-3 lack. Cardiovascular problems are a possibility — but rather more common are skin problems like itching, rashes, peeling, dryness, dandruff, and possibly hair loss. Fatigue, inflammatory problems like arthritis and swelling of joints, ringing in the ears, allergies and food sensitivities are others. Occasionally, low thyroid function can also occur.

The common omega-6 oils are mostly overused in the all-American diet, having been promoted as reducing blood cholesterol levels. The omega-3 oils do even better at reducing elevated blood cholesterol levels. The incorrect balance of oils can lead to reduced immune-system function. Excessive oil consumption can also promote cancer, if the oil is not protected from rancidity inside the body by taking extra vitamin E. Excess oil can worsen gout.

Vitamin K

Vitamin K is one of a number of factors that promote normal blood clotting. Symptoms of deficiency are easy bruising, nose bleeds or other hemorrhaging. You'll get plenty of vitamin K in vegetables such as dark green leafies and broccoli. You won't usually find vitamin K in supplements. You can get shorted in vitamin K by not eating vegetables, through malabsorption of fats, liver problems, celiac disease, trying to eat a no-fat diet, or by taking antibiotics. Taking yogurt can restart vitamin K production by intestinal bacteria.

Bioflavonoids

Bioflavonoids are especially useful in enhancing the effects of Vitamin C. The pulp of citrus fruits is especially rich in bioflavonoids. You can also take tablets. A one gram tablet gives you as much as one orange. Bioflavonoids help keep the walls of your small capillaries from breaking. Those who bruise easily or get nosebleeds may need additional bioflavonoids, vitamin C, or vitamin K.

Pangamic Acid

This non-vitamin nutrient, sometimes called vitamin B-15, appears to help promote good tissue oxygenation and tends to fortify the immune system. It is available as calcium pangamate, and the usual dosage runs 50 to 150 mg.

The Minerals

Unfortunately, the public does not have much experience with mineral supplementation. The only two minerals that have been emphasized much in the past are calcium and iron — two which answer the needs of women but not men. In supplementing with minerals, the risks of side effects can be far greater than with vitamins. To put it another way, the ranges of safe dosage are less than with vitamins. Only rarely will you want to be taking a mineral supplement in much greater amounts than the RDA, for there is too great a chance of interfering with other minerals. If you need to take two minerals that interfere with one another, you may avoid the interference problem by taking supplements of the two interfering minerals at a different time of day or on different days. If using supplements primarily for nutritional insurance (assuming there are no serious mineral deficiencies), a multimineral tablet will be adequate.

Magnesium

Although I've covered magnesium already, there is much more that is important. Deficiency causes health problems that develop insidiously and all sorts of stresses or bad habits cause loss of body magnesium stores. It's no surprise that many people get depleted of magnesium.

There are several possible interferences with other minerals. There is a three way interference between calcium, phosphorus and magnesium. Thus, if you have a diet of meat, milk, refined foods and phosphorus-loaded soft drinks, you'll be in trouble. Doesn't that sound a bit like the all-American diet?

Signs or symptoms that can suggest magnesium deficiency are: insomnia, tension, being overly keyed up, jumpiness at the slightest noise, anxiety, muscular twitching or tetany, tremors, convulsions, vertigo (dizziness), excessive sweating or body odor, depression, confusion or disorientation, memory impairment, apathy, paranoia, involuntary hand movements, difficulty in swallowing, asthma, angina, heart arrhythmia, congestive heart failure, stupor or coma, nystagmus (involuntary rapid oscillating eye movements), hallucinations (usually visual), etc. If you have a number of these signs, there is a good chance that you are magnesium deficient, or have a depletion of body stores. In some cases, the first overt signs of magnesium depletion can be changes in the electrocardiogram, a heart attack, or sudden cardiac death. Some drugs may contribute to depleting you of magnesium, such as antibiotics, diuretics, and digitalis.

The opposite problem, magnesium excess, can be seen in cases of kidney failure. It can also be seen with excessive supplementation with magnesium. The most likely symptoms would be lethargy, unexcitability and a slow heart rate.

The proper amount of magnesium supplementation you should get each day depends drastically on the type of life you lead and the foods you eat. If you have been on the all-American diet, you should add 200 to 300 mg. per day. If you have been on the all-American diet and living life in the fast lane, with assorted bad habits, you should add something like 500 mg. per day. If you eat whole foods and lead a fairly stress-free life, you may not need any extra magnesium. Along with magnesium supplementation, it's good to get 25 mg. per day vitamin B-6 to help the magnesium get into your cells. The usual magnesium supplements are magnesium oxide or dolomite. Dolomite has calcium, too, but sometimes has lead as well. If you take chelated magnesium, you won't need quite as much supplemental magnesium. The best absorbed magnesium supplement is probably magnesium aspartate. If you have digestive problems, especially low stomach acids, you'll especially need the chelated forms.

Calcium

Many Americans tend to get a poor balance of minerals from their diet. The excess salt that many consume tends to increase the loss of calcium through the urine. To make up for this loss, rather than supplementing heavily with calcium, which would then work against your magnesium status (through the calcium-phosphorus-magnesium interference), it is best to cut back on salt. The extra calcium would also work against your zinc and manganese status through another type of interference.

However, if you get too little calcium, you are setting yourself up for high blood pressure and a stroke, unless you cut down on your salt and get more magnesium in your diet (as would be found in a typical primitive diet).

Perhaps now you are beginning to see how complicated it gets when you have nutritional imbalances. But don't start worrying too much about balance. Your body can tolerate minor imbalances if you get enough of all the essential nutrients so that the regulatory mechanisms can work efficiently.

The RDA for calcium is 800 mg. per day. You should try to get that through cheese, yogurt, greens, tofu, beans, tortillas — preferably avoiding milk. However, if you are allergic to cheese or yogurt, you can expect to need calcium supplementation. Oyster shell, egg shell calcium or chelated calcium are probably the best supplements. If you take in 800 mg. of calcium, then you ought to get about 500 mg. magnesium. There appear to be considerable individual differences in calcium needs, some needing more like 1200 mg. per day. However, the apparent extra need for calcium may disappear when the rest of the diet is improved.

Sodium and Potassium

I'm covering these two together because of their mutual interference with one another. If you get too much sodium, it will adversely affect your potassium status, and vice versa. Refined foods that have salt added are good examples of what not to eat. They've lost their potassium and magnesium, and gained sodium, making them a one-way ticket to imbalance. If you are going to salt your food anyway, you might switch from using sodium chloride to using a salt that is a mixture of potassium chloride and sodium chloride. It is readily available in your supermarket.

A shortage of potassium will generally lead to muscle weakness. There are some people who appear to need a sizable sodium intake, just as there are others who can't tolerate much sodium without bloating up or getting high blood pressure. Those who work in a hot environment are likely to need extra sodium and other minerals.

Zinc and Copper

There is a strong mutual interference between these two trace elements. Since zinc supplementation has become popular, there have been numerous people who have driven their copper levels down. Note that large doses of vitamin C can also drive copper levels down. If you get much fructose, such as in corn sweeteners, your copper status will suffer. A diet of refined foods is seriously lacking in copper, but you might get enough copper if you have copper plumbing in your home. A lack of copper can contribute to numerous problems, including irregular heart beat, high blood cholesterol, ulcers and gout. Arthritis can result from either too little or too much copper, but there are other possible nutritional factors in arthritis.

The ideal ratio of zinc to copper in a supplement for someone in reasonable balance is about ten to one, but the ratio can vary between 7 and 15. In other words, a reasonable supplement might be 20 mg. zinc and 2 mg. copper. If you are depleted of both zinc and copper, you must take the zinc and copper supplements at different times of day for the best effect. Also, note that folic acid supplements can interfere with zinc absorption. Thus, if it is important that you get zinc supplementation, take zinc tablets a half-day apart from folic acid tablets.

White spots on your fingernails are the clearest sign of a need for more zinc. Supplementation with 30 to 50 mg. of zinc plus 25-50 mg. of vitam B-6 daily would be appropriate for most cases. Others with zinc deficiency, or extra need for zinc, are a bit harder to identify, but tell-tale signs are a history of eczema (a skin condition), slow maturation in young men, or prostate problems in older men. Therapeutic doses of zinc of 150 mg. are sometimes used, but don't appear necessary when vitamin B-6 is taken as well. The side effects of excess zinc dosage are most likely to be lethargy, nausea or diarrhea. A depressed immune system can occur from either too little or too much zinc.

Zinc is excellent for helping to rid the body of toxic metals, such as lead and cadmium.

Iron

Maintaining your iron status at a reasonable level gives you more physical energy.

Men don't tend to need much iron supplementation; the RDA of 10 mg. should be adequate for most. Women aged 15 to 50 need about twice as much. The supplement should be the *ferrous* form of iron, not the *ferric* form, which is useless. There are a number of different minerals that, in excess, will interfere with your iron status: manganese, zinc, cobalt, phosphorus and potassium. Vitamin C is very helpful in promoting iron absorption, as are copper and nickel. Oddly, excess copper works against iron. Heavy tea and coffee intake can work against iron absorption.

Manganese

Most Americans, as compared to people of the less developed nations, are low in manganese. The reason appears to be our methods of fertilizing the soil, which cause our vegetables to be short in manganese. The minerals that interfere with manganese status are calcium, potassium and phosphorus.

There can be subtle health problems that develop when you are short on manganese. Because manganese aids the utilization of B and C vitamins, someone short in manganese will find benefit in sizable doses of the B and C vitamins. A long-term manganese deficiency can contribute to diabetes or osteoporosis. It takes time to restore body manganese levels — years. Supplements aren't well retained by the body but are still worthwhile in the amount of 5 to 25 mg. per day. English-type tea is the richest dietary source of manganese.

Chromium

The typical American has low body stores of chromium. Chromium is extremely important for proper blood sugar regulation. Its lack is associated with atherosclerosis, hypoglycemia or diabetes. Eating sugar or taking sweet drinks tends to cause chromium loss through the urine. The phosphorus in milk tends to bind up and render useless the chromium in food.

Among chromium supplements, GTF-chromium is by far the most useful one, for it is well absorbed and utilized. A maintenance dose of GTF-chromium might have 50 mcg. elemental chromium, while a therapeutic dose would have 200 mcg. or more.

Selenium

It looks like selenium helps protect you from both cancer and heart disease. A safe and adequate dose of selenium is considered to be 50 to 200 micrograms. Selenium is toxic at levels of 500 to 1,000 micrograms daily.

Iodine

Iodine will be found in seafood, kelp, and in most multi-mineral supplement tablets. If you get too little iodine, it can lead to goiter. However, some people have a problem with even modest supplements of iodine, which may cause them to break out with acne.

Nickel, Vanadium, Molybdenum, Silicon, Fluorine, Boron, Arsenic and Tin

These trace elements have been found to be essential, but only in tiny amounts. You won't usually find them in supplement tablets, especially arsenic or fluorine (fluoride), since they are toxic at fairly low levels. You'll find a sufficient amount of these minerals in whole foods but not in refined foods.

Amino Acids

Additionally, many of the amino acids are becoming important in nutritional therapy for health problems. Thus phenylalanine is found helpful for pain or depression. Lysine supplementation can help prevent viruses from multiplying in your body. Tryptophan taken before bedtime can help some insomniacs. Glutamine supplements can help some alcoholics kick the habit. Tyrosine is being found useful, in conjunction with vitamins, in helping those hooked on cocaine avoid the blues after they quit. The dosages of amino acids used, several grams per day, are more than you could ever get from your food.

Once more, I must emphasize that you are playing Russian roulette with your long-term health when you eat refined foods, for you'll be cheated of both vitamins and minerals. The subtle physical and psychological ailments you develop will not seem to have much relation to your nutrient intakes, until after you eliminate the ailments by increasing nutrient intakes. On refined foods, for example, your body may no longer be able to regulate its mineral levels properly. You may absorb toxic metals, and/or end up with mineral imbalances — different imbalances in different people.

Beating The Odds

It would be easy to blame the medical profession for slowness to change, the legal profession for venality, the food industry for opportunism, the public for buying and eating junk (and expecting too much of medicine), or the government for its bureaucratic tangles. More fairly, we might blame the so-called civilized society which we seem to have evolved. Or, more basically, we might admit that we need to improve the way in which individuals relate to one another. As indicated previously, nutrition can influence our mental well-being, and thus our ability to relate to others amicably. However, many factors other than diet work against us. For instance, experiments have shown that noise makes people uncaring about their fellow man. Crowds and cities also have this effect. Still, we must reckon that the long-term dietary drift that has occurred contributes to a significant share of our interpersonal problems.

First let me summarize the dietary changes you need to protect your health:

1. Switch from fluid milk to fermented forms of milk, such as cheese or yogurt (preferably in low-fat and low-salt forms).

2. Switch from refined grains and sugars to whole grains and starches. These should include the bran (fiber) as well. Because of the limited shelf life of whole-grain flours, consider buying the grains and grinding them yourself on an inexpensive electric grain-grinder.

3. Cut back on most fats and oils, but get some omega-3 oil into your diet. Omega-3 oils are found richest in cold-water fish, and in food-grade linseed oil. (Other oils containing significant amounts of omega-3 are walnut, wheat germ, and soybean.) You can make excellent salad dressings with linseed oil. If you don't like fish, and insist on continuing a high fat diet, take EPA capsules.

4. Back away from food products that use refined grains and tend to be loaded with salt, fat and sugar.

5. If you are going to continue using a salt shaker, at least use a salt that is a mixture of potassium chloride and sodium chloride.

If you have a family history of heart disease, cancer, stroke or diabetes, you must be even more careful in your diet, perhaps getting additional salads and vegetables. Vitamin/mineral supplements can give an extra measure of protection.

Now let me summarize the general range of daily vitamin and mineral supplementation that you'll probably find optimal:

Vitamin A, 10,000 to 40,000 i.u. (Dosage in the upper part of the range should be accompanied by vitamin E and C supplements. Women who are pregnant must avoid sizable vitamin A doses.)

B-complex tablet, from RDA amounts up to a "B-50" tablet.

Extra folic acid, vitamin B-6 or pantothenic acid, as needed.

Vitamin C, 1,000 to 5,000 mg., preferably with some bioflavonoids.

Vitamin D, 200 i.u., but none if you get much sunshine.

Vitamin E, 100 to 400 i.u., in either the "d-alpha" or "mixed" tocopherol form.

Magnesium, 100 to 500 mg. supplementation, depending upon diet and lifestyle. Men need more than women.

Calcium, total daily intake of 800 mg., from both food and supplements.

Zinc, 10 to 30 mg.

Copper, 1 to 3 mg.

Iron, 10 mg. for men, and 18 mg. for women.

Manganese, 5 to 15 mg. Women planning to have children must make certain they get manganese.

Chromium, 50 to 200 micrograms, from GTF-chromium.

Selenium, 0 to 150 micrograms, depending upon diet and the region where you live.

The above figures assume that you don't have special health problems. Of course, dosages must be tailored to the individual situations, and therapeutic doses will be higher.

Not included in the supplement list are a number of ultra-trace elements which are also important. We have to depend upon a variety of whole foods for a source. Also, we must avoid taking an excess of supplements of the more common trace elements, because interferences may block absorption of ultra-trace elements.

Men need more in the way of supplements than women, partly on the basis of their greater weight. But men also need more, in proportion, of the antioxidants (vitamins A, C and E, and selenium) and certain minerals: magnesium, zinc and copper. Women tend to need more iron and calcium.

If you can practice a bit of nutritional self-discipline to overcome the innate tastes (for sugar, salt and fat) that lead us astray, and heed the lessons in this chapter about the problems of milk and refined foods, then you'll be well on your way to preventing health calamities in your life. As added insurance, at modest cost and effort, it is wise to get in the habit of taking vitamin and mineral supplements. You will also do well to encourage others around you to improve their nutritional habits. Hopefully, it will bring about better health and lower medical costs for all of us.

Here's to your optimum health!